MW01243597

THE CURSE OF OVARIAN CANCER

A CASE STUDY

Harvey Meredith, Ph.D.

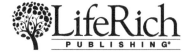

LifeRich PUBLISHING®

LifeRich Publishing is a registered trademark of The Reader's Digest Association, Inc.

LifeRich Publishing books may be ordered through booksellers or by contacting:

LifeRich Publishing
1663 Liberty Drive
Bloomington, IN 47403
www.liferichpublishing.com
844-686-9607

ISBN: 978-1-4897-4475-3 (sc)
ISBN: 978-1-4897-4476-0 (e)

Print information available on the last page.

LifeRich Publishing rev. date: 11/03/2022

In loving memory of Celeste, the most perfect lady I have ever known, I miss her terribly. (2/16/28-12/25/21)

CONTENTS

PREFACE

In the thirteen years I knew Celeste, we never had a disagreement. She was the most compatible person I ever knew. She was never moody or outwardly depressed. She was always upbeat, positive, and busy with activities of her interests. Even when struggling with cancer treatments, she managed to maintain a favorable outlook and was always pleasant. She was among the most honest people I have ever known. I could predict how Celeste would come down on most topics. She made decisions based on her interests and those which met her character. She was likely the most determined person I have ever known. Persistence was a quality she owned.

Celeste had a long list of diverse activities that she loved. One was spending time at South Padre Island. The beach and the water were a special attraction for her. She attacked the waves as a teenager. When knocked down, she sprang up laughing at herself. Her last trip was October of 2021.

She enjoyed cruises to many places around the world. Her love included daily dips in the pool when possible. She ensured a pool would not be distant and added a swimming pool to her homes. For the last 13 years she lived in an association with a pool and she enjoyed aerobic water classes at the YMCA pools. She had traveled extensively prior to our meeting, but her desire for new adventures had not declined.

Celeste took piano lessons at age 16, working in a drug store to pay for the lessons and became an accomplished pianist. She could play most any music beautifully. Celeste had taken up art working with water colors, acrylics, lithography and mosaics. She borrowed $1,000 from her father and put herself through college. Her major was mechanical engineering and architecture, initially. She ended up in architecture, a five-year college program and worked a career as an engineering draftsman for oil companies. Celeste was fearful of heights so after she retired, she took flying lessons to become a pilot to overcome this fear.

She was a Life Master in the bridge world. She had played in tournaments around the state to gain the gold and silver points required to become a Life Master. One of her great enjoyments was playing competitive bridge every Monday afternoon until it was stopped due to COVID-19. She was a vociferous reader, making trips to the library and always checking out three or four books each time. Celeste loved movie theatres, Netflix, and library movies. She worked the crossword puzzle from the daily newspaper at the breakfast table, often finishing in record time with perfect engineering drawing lettering, in ink. Then, she would casually place the puzzle in the trash receptacle. She completed the last crossword puzzle on December 17, 2021.

She did not have a large wardrobe of clothes but she could put together combinations so that she looked classy. She never left the house without looking spiffy, not even to the grocery store. She always told me that you never know who you might see! Even when wearing something like levies, she would always top it off with a decorative addition to make her dress special.

Her big love was flowers and plants. She always grew a huge display of plants of all description, many unusual tropical plants that needed to be overwintered in the garage. She tended the flowers herself, often working outside until darkness closed her day. She knew the names of the plants, even the most exotic ones by both the common and scientific name. When her plants were blooming, the first activity each day was to go outside and pick assorted flowers for a daily arrangement. She relied on the grocery store to supplement her flower arrangements out of season, but she always had flowers throughout the house.

When Celeste bought her last home in 2010, at age 81, she did not like the darkness in the dinette area. She decided she wanted a double window in the wall on the side of the house without windows. The contractor who built the house lived two houses away and was on the architect committee for the Association. He reviewed the project and determined if the bricks were removed in the wall, the wall would come crumbling down. Celeste put his comments on the back burner and contacted a skillful contractor who had rebuild her deck with Timber Tech, an artificial wood, who had done a marvelous job. She had previously had the same fellow rearrange the plumbing in her bathroom and install California closets. This fellow told Celeste that it would be no problem and undertook the project. When completed, the kitchenette was well lighted with two large windows that looked as if they had been part of the original house. A reminder of her determination!

The string on one of the venetian blinds in a three-panel window broke. After all efforts to repair the string failed, Celeste went to the phone and ordered blinds and when they arrived, she hung them herself. She said, they told me how to measure them and I placed the order. This she accomplished when she was 91 years old.

Celeste and I considered each other our most precious friends. There was nothing either of us would not have done for the other. When Celeste was diagnosed with cancer, we attacked it together. Celeste never had a cancer treatment without the presence of both of us. I missed one doctor's appointment, otherwise, I was at her side for doctor's appointments as well.

Celeste was diagnosed by our family doctor on June 26, 2019. It was diagnosed as Uterine Papillary Serous Carcinoma (USC), Stage III. It is a type II cancer, an aggressive variant of endometrial cancer. It accounts for less than 10 percent of all endometrial cancers and 80 percent of endometrial cancer related deaths.

Celeste accepted the diagnosis of ovarian cancer with a will to fight it as no other battle in her life. She had always been so careful with her health and her diet. She never drank coffee or tea and enjoyed oatmeal and salads most every day. She never asked, "Why Me" when she was stricken with such a tragic disease as a rare deadly ovarian cancer. The cancer, has few if any survivors. Celeste was in such great physical condition (she was at the gym five days a week), she felt confident she would be a survivor. Life was so precious to her. She had been a member of the YMCA and other gyms for over 30 years. She was strong and healthy. She would handle two 10-pound weights on the weight bench and exercise for long periods of time along with her regular exercise routine. There was no family history of cancer. She carried 128 pounds on a five-foot, seven-inch frame, and she was diligent about keeping her weight constant. She continued her gym schedule after being diagnosed and during cancer treatments.

I was proudest of Celeste for the manner in which she took on the curse of her cancer. It was a courage and conviction with fearless dedication. She was so determined to do everything humanly possible to defeat the cancer and she was relentless to ensure the cancer and treatments would not interfere with living a near normal life and enjoy each day to the fullest. Outwardly, one would never have guessed what she was experiencing. Her Herculean character was forever on display as never before. She always maintained a pleasant outlook and her spirits were elevated.

After completing a total of 22 chemo treatments in two different series, the cancer doctor in charge of her cancer treatments, decided to try different chemicals, which proved to be a disaster. When the chemicals failed to control the cancer and damaged her heart and liver, the cancer doctor decided to stop all treatments and turn Celeste over to Hospice.

It was a bitter pill to swallow. It was a cruel, cold, and unjust decision on the part of this doctor. Celeste looked healthy, the same as she always looked. How could a doctor issue such a death warrant to someone who had so much life? Celeste had been a perfect patient and did everything that was asked of her. She handled chemo well. She had completed two series of the same chemo chemicals and her cancer level, CA-125 (cancer antibody), the cancer marker for ovarian cancer, dropped to "normal" at the end of both treatment series. The cancer rebounded in both cases. Chemo can be given up to six series. Celeste handled the chemo treatments well and they were successful against the recurring invasion of ovarian cancer. The cancer was too aggressive to go into remission. Additional chemo would have been a life extension to someone who looked at life as such a precious gift. Why the cancer doctor decided to try chemicals that had dangerous side effects and which were not successful against the ovarian cancer cells, cannot be explained. Celeste was able to live a near normal life with the chemo treatments. Continuing the chemo treatments would have kept Celeste with us for a much longer time. The chemicals selected by this doctor damaged her heart and kidneys. Celeste was a young 93 at the time. The dose rate, wrong treatment or some other incompetence, must accept the blame for her death.

I never fully realized how precious Celeste was or how much she truly meant to me. I regret that I could not tell her daily how much I loved and admired her.

Chapter 1

WHAT IS CANCER?

Have a caring heart, a smile that never fades and a touch that never hurts.

----unknown

Cancer is a disease in which abnormal cells divide uncontrollably and destroy body tissue. Cancer is caused by changes in DNA. Most cancer-causing DNA changes occur in sections of the DNA called genes. There are 20,000-25,000 genes per cell. These changes are referred to as genetic changes.

In the U.S. in 2020, cancer was the second leading cause of death behind heart disease. A total of 602,350 lives were lost to cancer, 52.7% were males.

In 2022, 609,360 people are estimated to die from cancer in the U.S. Lung and bronchus cancer account for the most deaths. Colorectal cancer is the second most common death due to cancer in the U.S.

Cancer can start almost anywhere in the body which is made up of an estimated 37.2 trillion cells. Normally, human cells grow and multiply through a controlled process called cell division, to form new cells, as the body needs them. When cells grow old or become damaged, they are replaced, and new cells take their place. This process is ongoing at all times.

Different types of genes in the body have different jobs. The nucleus of the cell is the control center. Inside the nucleus are chromosomes.

Normally, each cell in the human body has 23 pairs of chromosomes or 46 total. Half come from the female and half from the male parents. Genes contain long strings of DNA (deoxyribonucleic acid) which contain coded messages that control the cell function. This is the genetic information that a parent passes on to biological children.

Each gene contains an instruction that directs the function within the cell to produce a protein or a different type of molecule called RNA (ribonucleric acid). Together proteins and RNA control the cell. They decide what sort of cell it will be, function and when it will divide or die.

When the system is functioning properly, genes control the growth and reproduction in an orderly and controlled way. Sometimes a change occurs in the genes when a cell divides. This is called a mutation. It means a gene has been damaged, lost or copied twice. Sometimes mutations mean the cell no longer understands its instruction and starts to grow out of control.

Cancer cells are cells that have gone wrong. They no longer respond to many of the signals that control cellular growth and death. Cancer cells originate within tissues and as they divide and grow, they deviate from normalcy even more. Over time these cells become increasingly resistant to the normal controls of cells. Cancer cells divide more rapidly than normal cells and become less dependent on signals from other cells. Cancer cells actually evade programmed cell death. Normally, their multiple abnormalities would make the prime target for apoptosis (death).

Hundreds of genes control the process of cell division in normal cells. Normally, there is a balance between the activity of those genes that promote cell proliferation and those that suppress it. Genes signal when damaged cells should undergo apoptosis.

Cells become cancerous after mutations occur in the various genes that control cellular proliferation. The Cancer Genome Project determined that most cancer cells possess 60 or more mutations. Because of the large number of mutations that occur in cells to become cancerous, the timeframe for initiation of cancer to tumor stage is not elaborated upon. The task, prevent such mutations and determine which mutations are responsible for development into cancer.

Different cancers have different mutational signatures. Cancer related mutations inactivate the genes that suppress cell proliferation or those that signal the need for apoptosis. Tumor suppressor genes, normally function like brakes on proliferation, and both copies within a cell must be mutated in order for uncontrolled cell division to occur. It says, development of normal cells into cancer cells is not an easy or quick transition.

Gene mutations accumulate over time as a result of independent events. The path to cancer involves multiple steps. Cancer may be viewed as a microevolutionary process.

When a mutation gives a cancer cell a growth advantage, it can make more copies of itself than a normal cell. Its offspring can outperform the noncancerous counter parts in the competition for resources. A second mutation may provide the cancer cell with yet another reproductive advantage, and in turn intensifies the competitive advantage further. The process continues with every new mutation. Such is the driving force in the evolution of living things.

In the early stages of cancer, tumors are typically benign and are confined within the normal boundaries of a tissue. As tumors grow and become malignant, they gain the ability to break through these boundaries and invade adjoining tissues.

When the orderly process breaks down at the cellular level, abnormal or damaged cells grow and multiply. These cells may form tumors, which appear as lumps of tissue. Tumors can be cancerous or benign.

Cancerous tumors spread into, or invade, nearby tissues and can travel to distant places in the body to form new tumors, a process called metastasis. Cancerous tumors are called malignant tumors.

Benign tumors do not spread into, or invade, nearby tissues. When removed, benign tumors normally don't grow back. Benign tumors can be large and need to be removed.

Cancer cells and normal cells differ in many ways. Normal cells are controlled by signals that tell cells when to stop dividing or die, a process known as programmed cell death, apoptosis. Cancer cells grow in the absence of signals, uncontrollably. They can invade nearby areas and spread to different areas of the body. Normal cells stop growing when encountering other cells, and most normal cells do not roam around in the body.

Cancer cells have the ability to form new blood vessels to supply tumors with oxygen and nutrients and remove waste products from tumors.

The immune system of the body protects against infections, viruses, and multiple functions detrimental to the body. The immune system normally eliminates damaged or abnormal cells. Cancer cells hide from the immune system and survive. Cancer cells trick the immune system into helping cancer cells survive and grow. Thus, cancer cells can make the immune system protect cancer cells and cancerous tumors instead of attacking them.

The cancer cells can cause changes in the chromosomes, such as duplication and deletion of chromosome parts. Some cancer cells have double the number of chromosomes as a normal cell.

Cancer cells can utilize different kinds of nutrients and can make nutrients differently than normal cells allowing cancer cells to grow more quickly.

Cancer is called a genetic disease because cancer is caused by changes in the genes that control the way cells function, especially growth and cell division.

Genetic changes can occur in many ways. Errors occur in cell division, damage to DNA caused by harmful substances in the environment, such as chemicals in smoke and sun ultraviolet rays. Genetic changes continue with a person's cancer, even within the tumor itself. Cancer is unchecked cell growth.

The body normally eliminates cells with damaged DNA before they can turn cancerous. The body's ability to destroy damaged cells declines with age, resulting in a higher risk of cancer later in life. This also says, as you age one must pay more attention to factors that not only cause cancer but measures one must take to protect against cancer as best it is understood.

Cancer starts with changes in one cell or a small group of cells. Cells produce signals to control how much and how often the cells divide. If any signals are faulty or missing, cells may start to grow and multiply to form a lump called a tumor. A primary tumor is where the cancer starts. For a cancer to form, changes take place within the genes of a cell or group of cells. Cancer is uncontrolled cell division.

The genetic changes that contribute to cancer tend to affect three main types of genes: proto-oncogenes, tumor suppressor genes, and DNA repair genes. Proto-oncogenes are involved in normal cell growth and cell division. When these genes are altered and become more active than normal, they may become cancer-causing genes or oncogenes. This change allows cells to grow and survive, when they should normally die.

Tumor suppressor genes are involved in controlling cell division. Cells with certain alterations in tumor suppressor genes may divide in an uncontrolled manner.

DNA repair genes are involved in fixing damaged DNA. Cells with mutations in these genes tend to develop additional mutations in other genes and changes in their chromosomes, as duplications and deletions of chromosome parts. These combined activities may initiate cancerous cells.

A cancer that has spread from the place of initiation to another place in the body is called metastatic cancer. The process by which the cancer cells spread is called metastasis. The metastatic cancer is the same as the original cancer. Under a microscope, metastatic cancer cells generally look the same as cells of the original cancer. They have molecular features in common, such as presence of specific chromosome changes.

There are tissue changes that are not cancer. **Hyperplasia** – cells within a tissue multiply faster than normal cells and extra cells build up. The cells look the same as normal cells. Hyperplasia is caused by several factors or conditions; one might be constant irritation.

Dysplasia – is a more advanced condition then hyperplasia. With dysplasia there is a buildup of extra cells but the cells look abnormal. In general, the more abnormal the cells and tissue looks under a microscope, the greater chance cancer will form. An example of dysplasia is an abnormal mole (dysplastic nevus) that forms on the skin. A dysplastic nevus can turn into melanoma.

Carcinoma in situ is an even more advanced condition. It is sometimes referred to as Stage 0 cancer. It is not a cancer, as the cells are not abnormal, and they do not invade nearby tissue. Because they could become cancerous, they are usually treated.

There are more than 100 types of cancers. A type of cancer is usually named for the organs or tissues where the cancer forms. Cancers may be described by the type of cell that formed them, such as epithelial cell or a squamous cell. There are categories of cancers that begin in specific types of cells as:

Carcinoma – the most common type of cancer, formed by epithelial cells that cover the inside and outside surfaces of the body. There are many types of epithelial cells, which often have a column-like shape when viewed under a microscope. Carcinomas that begin in different epithelial cell types have specific names.

Adenocarcinoma – a cancer that forms in epithelial cell types that produce fluids or mucus.

Epithelial -about 90 percent of ovarian cancers are epithelial tumors which originate in the thin layers of tissue covering the outside of the ovaries.

Each cancer gets its name from the point of its origination. Ovarian cancer originates in the ovaries. Early-stage ovarian cancer rarely causes any symptoms. Advanced stage ovarian cancer may cause few and nonspecific symptoms.

About 90 percent of ovarian cancers are epithelial (the thin layer of tissue covering the ovary). Ovarian cancer is most common in women 50-60 years of age and older.

Chapter 1a

UTERINE SEROUS CARCINOMA (USC)

Work is about a search for daily meaning as well as daily bread.

----unknown

Endometrial (uterine) cancer (EC) is the fourth most commonly diagnosed malignancy and the seventh most common cause of cancer deaths in women in the U.S. Endometrial cancer involves malignant (cancer) cells from the tissues of the endometrium (the lining of the uterus). The endometrium, the hollow, muscular organ in a woman's pelvis, is where a fetus grows and develops. Approximately 65,950 new cases will be diagnosed and 12,550 EC –related deaths will occur in 2022, marking increases in incidence and mortality. Worldwide, EC is the fourth most common tumor type and accounts for 5 percent of all cancer cases and 2 percent of all cancer deaths. EC's highest incidence occurs in North America and Northern Europe, especially in the developed countries (1,2) This is also the area of the world where the highest consumption of milk and dairy products occurs.

Uterine serous carcinoma (USC), although rare, is the most lethal of uterine cancers. This is the type cancer Celeste had. It is an aggressive variant of endometrial cancer that has not been well characterized. It accounts for less than 10 percent of all endometrial cancers and 80 percent of endometrial cancer-related deaths. (3,4) It has an extremely low survival rate, if any. I am not certain, and I don't believe anyone really knows, if there are any survivors beyond 5 years from USC, especially if diagnosed in stage III or IV. It has distinct molecular features and pathogenic pathways compared with other uterine cancer types.

A combination of surgery, chemotherapy and radiotherapy is the primary strategy for USC and this has been the standard treatment for 30 years.

Using the Boklman's 1983 model, EC is broadly classified based on histopathologic features into two categories, type I and type II. They differ in incidence, prognosis, epidemiology, molecular pathology and clinical behavior. (5)

Type I tumors account for about 90 percent of all ECs. This cancer displays a well-differentiated endometrioid histological phenotype and, compared with type II tumors, has a favorable prognosis, earlier onset (diagnosis) and a higher 5-year survival rate. (6)

Type I tumors are typically associated with obesity, and usually develop from an environment of endometrial hyperplasia resulting from excess exposure to either endogenous (inside of body) or exogenous (outside of body) estrogen. (6,7) Milk is an excellent source of estrogen as pregnant cows have high levels of estrogen in the placenta, especially in the later months of pregnancy. Pregnant cows are milked until late in pregnancy.

Type II tumors, such as serous carcinoma, are characterized by poorly differentiated histology and deep migration and invasion. Type II tumors are typically diagnosed in women 70 years or older, in stage III or IV, and have a poor prognosis, high recurrence frequency, and very low 5-year survival rate, if any, compared to type I. Type II tumors lack estrogen/progesterone receptors and do not respond to hormonal treatments. (7)

Among the type II tumors, uterine serous carcinoma (USC) is the most common subtype. As was noted earlier, this highly aggressive variant accounts for only 10 percent or less of all ECs but 80 percent of all EC-associated deaths. The risk of metastasis and recurrence of USC does not depend on primary tumor size or grade. This trait contributes to the low survival rate.

Because of poor patient survival, high recurrence rates, coupled with relatively low percentage of patients, development of targeted therapies specific to USC pathway aberrations has not been a high enough priority. Conducting studies that focus solely on this rare subtype has not been challenged sufficiently and ultimate strategies have not been developed. (4)

Type II ECs, especially USC, have a complex papillary or glandular architecture, which is similar to serous papillary ovarian carcinoma. (8,9) USC is commonly considered to be derived from its putative precursor, endometrial intraepithelial cancer. Endometrial glandular dysplasia has been proposed as a USC precursor as well (10,11).

In type II EC, the predominant alteration is TP53 gene, accounting for about 95 percent of cases and plays essential roles in almost all of the disease's stages, especially the early stage. (12) If there was a way to monitor TP53 gene, might this be a way to diagnose early-stage USC? USC has been found to harbor a 60 percent TP53 gene mutation rate.

Apparently, there are problems in interpretation of staining results and this factor needs further extensive evaluations. (13)

Targeted therapy for USC lags behind that of other cancer types. Due to the rarity of USC, few tests are specifically designed for USC patient cohorts. The most altered molecule in USC is p53 and the p53-associated signaling pathways are promising clinical targets. Currently, therapies targeting the p53 pathway focus on either restoring wild-type p53, "correcting" mutated p53 activities, or targeting the downstream effect of p53. (14)

USC studies are lacking due to its rare occurrence and the lack of animal models for the disease. Development of treatments for this cancer is far behind those for other cancers. Compared to all endometrial cancers, the number of USC patients is relatively small but accounts for such a high percentage of fatalities. This factor alone should ignite a challenge and be highly supported with the best research tools. Because of the aggressive features, poor prognosis, and extremely high recurrence rate (80 percent or better), all contribute to the increase of USC-related deaths every year. This is the most-deadly of all uterine cancers, perhaps one of the most-deadly of all cancers, and it is poorly understood. A cure is in the far distant future.

Pathogenesis and Clinical Management of Uterine Serous Carcinoma. (https://wwwlmdpi.com/2072-6694/12/3/686/htm

References:

1. Charo, L.M., Plaxe, S.C. Recent advances in endometrial cancer: A review of key clinical trials from 2015 to 2019. *F1000Reserch 2019, 8.*
2. Siegel, R.L., Miller, K.D., Jemal, A. Cancer statistics, 2019. *CA Cancer J. Clin.* 2019, 69, 7-34.
3. Group, S.G.O.C.P.E.E.W. Endometrial cancer: A review and current management strategies: Part II. *Gynecol. Oncol.* 2014, 134, 393-402.
4. Moore, K.N.; Fader, A.N. Uterine papillary serous carcinoma. *Clin. Obstet. Gyneco*l. 2011, 54, 278-291.
5. Creasman, W.T., Eddy, G.L. Recent advances in endometrial cancer. *Semin. Surg. Oncol.* 1990, 6, 339-342.
6. Saso, S. et.al. Endometrial cancer. *BMJ* 2011, 343, d3954.
7. Amant,F. et.al. Endometrial cancer. Lancet 2005, 366, 491-505.
8. Zheng, W.; Chambers, S.K. Histopathology of endometrial hyperplasia and endometrial carcinoma. An update by Dr. LC Horn et. al. in Annals of Diagnostic Pathology 2007;11:297-311. *Ann. Diagn. Pathol.* 2008, 12, 231232.
9. Nakayama, K. et.al. Endometrial serous carcinoma: Its molecular characteristics and histology-specific treatment strategies. *Cancers* 2012, 4,799-807.
10. Zheng, W. et.al. Endometrial glandular dysplasia: A newly defined precursor lesion of uterine papillary serous Carcinoma. Part I: Morphologic features. *Int. J. Surg. Pathol.* 2004, 12, 207-223.
11. Fadare, O.; Zheng, W. Endometrial Glandular Dysplasia (EmGD): Morphologically and biologically distinctive putative precursor lesions of Type II endometrial cancers. *Diagn. Pathol.* 2008,3,6.
12. La Gallo, M.; Bell, D.W. The emerging genomic landscape of endometrial cancer. *Clin. Chem.* 2014,60.98-110.
13. Alkushi, A; et.al. Interpretation of p53 immunoreactivity in endometrial carcinoma: Establishing a clinically relevant cut-off level. Int. J. Gynecol. *Pathol.* 2004,23,129-137.
14. Blandino, G; Di Agostino, S. New therapeutic strategies to treat human cancers expressing mutant p53 proteins. *J. Exp. Clin. Cancer Rev.* 2018,37,30.

Chapter 2

INTRODUCTION TO OVARIAN CANCER

The Lord said to the brethren, go and celebrate. A monk rewriting a document miscopied or misinterpreted and copied "celibate". (For that, many have struggled with themselves far too long!)

----unknown

Cancer is a disease involving dynamic changes in the genome. It is daunting in the breadth and scope of its diversity, spanning genetics, cell and tissue biology, pathology, and response to therapy.

Ovarian cancer has been described as an obsessive tumor and its home is the abdominal cavity and beyond. It is difficult to treat and its destructive nature has no limits. It changes the lives of its victims forever. Ovarian cancer destroys a women's health and steals her dignity. It will strike one woman in 78 or 1.3 percent in the U.S. and 1 in 108 women will die with ovarian cancer. It is most common in ages above 50 but teenage girls and women in their early twenties have had ovarian cancer, although extremely rare. Patients pay a horrific price. Those who survive advanced ovarian cancer, do so with unspeakable suffering.

Ovarian cancer is a deadly gynecological cancer. The tumor immune microenvironment (time) plays a pivotal role in ovarian cancer development. The length of time to develop ovarian cancer is not known. At the beginning, apparently it is slow. Dr. Susan Love has been quoted; "It takes 100 days for one cell to double and become two." Most breast cancers have been present for 8-10 years by the time one feels the smallest lump.

Symptoms are not readily discernable for ovarian cancer and diagnosis in late stages, occurs far too often. Symptoms masquerade as other problems; gastrointestinal disorders as an example. There are no early symptoms for ovarian cancer. Constipation, and reduced appetite due to bloating are perhaps the first and most notable and consistent symptoms. Bloating is caused by the liquid accumulation in the area above the stomach under the rib cage. Another symptom may include frequent urination. These symptoms should not be overlooked. There is no screening for ovarian cancer. Women with these symptoms may be in Stage III or IV before they are first diagnosed with ovarian cancer. Malignant (cancerous) cells in the biopsy of tissues of the ovary, confirm ovarian cancer. Ovarian cancer is the leading cause of death from all gynecological cancers. It is the fifth leading cause of cancer related deaths among women in the U.S.

Over 22,000 women in the U.S. will be diagnosed with ovarian cancer in one year. Ovarian cancer has the reputation as being one of the most difficult diseases to diagnose. It is also the most lethal of all gynecologic malignancies. Women who delay childbirth past their thirties or women who have no children are the most vulnerable. Women who have used birth control pills for at least five continuous years seem to have greatly reduced ovarian cancer. Women who have a complete hysterectomy, removal of fallopian tubes and both ovaries, will have a greatly reduced probability of ovarian cancer.

Women who take estrogen hormone treatments without the progesterone hormone, have a greater risk of ovarian cancer. Women with family histories of breast and ovarian cancer, also have a higher risk of ovarian cancer. Fertility drugs apparently do not increase the risk of ovarian cancer. The older the patient, the greater risk of ovarian cancer. Only about 14 percent of ovarian cancers are genetically linked.

Because of the late diagnosis, ovarian cancer patients will have extensive metastases in the abdominal cavity. Surgery is often recommended at the beginning of the treatment process. Although, that may be changing, likely due to the extensive surgery and the disruption of the body from the complex surgeries. Some advocate chemo treatments first to reduce the intensity of surgery which might occur later. Even though chemo treatments are effective, the recurrence rate is 80 percent or possibly higher when diagnosed in Stage III or IV.

Radiation and surgery for cancer are more than a hundred years old. Chemo therapy has been used for over 70 years, dating to the late 1940s. The two chemicals used in chemo treatments, Carboplatin and Paclitaxel (Taxol), have been used since the mid-90s.

Determining the process of how a cell becomes malignant or how long the process takes is not known. It is also not known how long the cancer cells may have been active before diagnoses. The process leading to the formation of malignant cells may involve years, possibly a decade or longer. Since there is no early way to identify malignant ovarian cancer cells, their progress is not noticed until the tumor makes itself known by one or more symptoms noted earlier. Fallopian tube cancers are identical to ovarian cancers and are treated the same. The ovary and the thin membrane that lines the interior of the abdomen, the peritoneal, are derived from the embryo's genital ridge. Peritoneal cancers and ovarian cancers are identical visibly and microscopically.

High-grade Serous Carcinoma is a common type of ovarian cancer that accounts for 75 percent of epithelial cancers. Many high-grade serous ovarian carcinomas (HGSOC), originate as a small tumor in the epithelium of fallopian tubes.

Uterine Serous Carcinoma (Celeste's cancer), is a rare subtype of endometrial cancer that behaves aggressively, with high risk. It represents less than 10 percent of all uterine cancers, although, it accounts for 80 percent of the deaths for endometrial cancer.

The median overall survival for patients with high-grade serous ovarian carcinoma is less than 40 months. Median – midpoint, an equal number above and below, meaning that 50 percent of the deaths occur less than 40 months following diagnosis. Celeste made it only to 30 months.

High-grade serous carcinoma cells and tissue viewed under a microscope appear highly abnormal compared to healthy cells and tissue. Tumor cells organize abnormally and grow quickly. High-grade serous ovarian carcinomas are classified as Grade 3. "Serous" meaning that the tumor arose from the serous membrane in the epithelial layer in the abdominopelvic cavity.

Recent studies indicate that high-grade carcinoma that originate with a primary tumor in the fallopian tubes, take as average of 6.5 years to reach the ovaries, after which they spread to other areas quickly. Taking the length of time to travel the relative short distance from the fallopian tubes to the ovaries, cancer cell development is likely a long process.

Advanced stage carcinomas generally spread to the peritoneum (the lining of the organs of the pelvis and abdomen) first, which can lead to fluid buildup in the peritoneal cavity, referred to as bloating. The fluid is called ascites, caused by metastasizing cancer cells.

The peritoneal produces the ascitic fluid. This fluid is normal, but cancer causes the peritoneum to produce too much of this fluid, called malignant ascites. It often is a sign of advanced cancer. This malignant ascites is caused by cancer that has spread to the lining of the organs inside the abdomen. It can happen when cancer spreads to the liver. Ascites build-up may occur with a vast array of cancers including breast, colon, gastrointestinal tract cancers as stomach and intestinal, ovarian and fallopian tube cancer, pancreatic and uterine cancer.

The ascites fluid build-up may cause weight gain, shortness of breath, abdominal swelling, feeling full quickly (satiety), sense of being full, bloating, sense of heaviness, constipation leading to hemorrhoids, fatigue, and loss of appetite. Care with any of the above symptoms is referred to as palliative care or supportive care.

Paracentesis is the term used when a needle is inserted into the abdomen to remove fluid (peritoneal fluid) for testing and/or to relieve bloating. The collected fluid is then analyzed. A liter to several liters may be removed each time.

A series of functional capabilities are acquired by human cells from normalcy to neoplastic states. Capabilities that are crucial to malignant tumors have been developed by Hanahan and Weisman. They envision eight distinct hallmark capabilities.

1. **Self-Sufficiency in Growth Signals**. Normal cells require inherent signals before they can proliferate. No normal cell can divide in the absence of such stimulatory signals. The hallmark of a cancer cell is its ability to generate its own growth signals, thereby initiating growth independent of the processes dictating the proliferation of the normal cell.

2. **Evading growth suppressors.** There are multiple anti-proliferative signals that operate within normal tissue that are responsible for normal tissue stability. By a number of mechanisms, some of which are not well understood, a cancer cell is able to evade these antiproliferative signals with ease.

3. **Resisting cell death**. Apoptosis (death) is programmed cell death, and this process of self-immolation is inherent in all normal cells. An acquired resistance to apoptosis is a unique quality in all cancer cells and confers on such cells an unfortunate immortality.

4. **Enabling replicative immortality.** The three acquired capabilities (growth signal autonomy, insensitivity to antigrowth signals, and resistance to apoptosis) lead to an uncoupling of a cell's growth program from signals in its environment. This causes the development of vast cell populations that eventually constitute a visible tumor.

5. **Sustained Angiogenesis.** The oxygen and nutrients supplied through blood vessels are necessary for cell function and survival. Angiogenesis is the process whereby new blood vessels are generated; feeding tumors with new blood vessels is absolutely necessary if cancer cells are to proliferate and a tumor is to grow.

6. **Tissue Invasion and Metastasis**. The capacity for invasion and metastasis enables cancer cells to escape the primary tumor site and invade other organs. This process can occur through the bloodstream, through lymphatic drainage, or, as is so frequently seen in ovarian cancer, by direct extension into organs within the abdominal cavity. The capacity, for metastatic spread of a cancer, is an extremely complex mechanism and remains a mystery.

7. **Reprogramming cellular metabolism.** An elaboration of #5 above

8. **Avoiding immune destruction.** Being able to avoid the natural immunity systems existing in a normal environment, are critical to the survival of cancer cells.

Cancer is a formidable and terrifying opponent. In view of what is known about cancer and how it operates, current treatment procedures appear feeble and almost ineffective against such a frightful foe. Research has yet to intercept malignant cell proliferation at the signaling pathway. To know how cancer operates is a start. The more information gathered about the complexity of cancer the more distant a cure appears.

The above paragraph must be reread and studied for it defines the extreme difficulty man encounters in getting the upper hand in treatment of cancer and ultimately finding a cure.

So little is known about the origin of cancer of the ovary. It is the damage to the ovary at ovulation that may be a contributing factor to the genesis of this cancer. Each month an explosion occurs in the ovary as the egg is released, following the rupture of the ovarian cyst that releases the egg. The cells that line the outermost part of the ovary, epithelial cells, proliferate to repair damage on the surface of the ovary. This action could be repeated monthly for over 30 years. Women for the most part do not ovulate during pregnancy, during the time they are breast feeding the child and while on birth control pills. Several pregnancies early in adult life, therefore, may be a protection against ovarian cancer.

Ovulation is the release of an egg from one of the two ovaries, although the exact timing may vary. In preparation of ovulation, the lining of the uterus, or endometrium, thickens. The pituitary gland in the brain stimulates one of the ovaries to release an egg. Ovulation usually occurs 10-16 days prior to menstruation.

The egg is released at about day 14 of a 28-day menstrual cycle. The egg travels out of the ovary and is taken up by the fallopian tube. As the fallopian tube is not attached to the ovary, the fallopian tube collects the egg from the abdominal cavity. After the release, the egg has about 12-24 hours to be fertilized by sperm in the fallopian tube.

Usually, one egg (oocyte) is released by the ovary during the menstrual cycle, with each ovary taking an alternate turn in releasing an egg. A female baby is born with all the eggs that she will ever have in her lifetime, and there are quite a few. At age 30, a woman might have 100,000-150,000 eggs. At age 35, she may have 80,000 and at the age of 40, 25,000-10,000.

A complex interaction between the pituitary gland in the brain, the ovaries and the uterus coordinate to create the perfect environment for ovulation to occur, for the sperm and egg to meet and for the fertilized egg to implant itself in the uterus. The part of the brain called the hypothalamus controls ovulation and the release of hormones during the menstrual cycle.

Birth control pills prevent ovulation. This is a protection against ovarian cancer if the birth control pills are taken for at least five consecutive years. Women who have children early in life and continue to give birth and nurse children, may ovulate only a few dozen times in their lifetime. Ovarian cancer is almost absent in this group of women. By this discussion, a woman on birth control pills during most of her premenopausal years, should have equal protection.

The relationship between talcum powder and ovarian cancer is of interest. A pathologist at Johns Hopkins University by the name of Donald Woodruff proposed that the granules from talcum powder get into the abdomen via the vagina, cervical canal, uterine cavity, and fallopian tubes. Microscopic slides of patients with ovarian cancer, quite often will have large, calcified granules called psammoma bodies or calcospherites. The question, how does the talc powder get inside the vagina and how much would it take to cause a problem? Are these calcified granules formed naturally without the presence of talc? Is talc really the factor causing these calcified granules?

The Lynch Syndrome, the hereditary nonpolyposis colorectal cancer (HNPCC), is associated with a higher risk for ovarian cancer. Women who live in tropical climates have a lower rate of ovarian cancer. Could this be related to a higher level of vitamin D? They would be spending a lot of time in the out-of-doors and exposed to sunshine, the Vitamin D source. The energy of the ultraviolet sun rays converts the D2 in the skin to D3, the available form of Vitamin D. Ultraviolet light is a short-wave radiation and does not penetrate clothing. It must strike bare skin. If vitamin D is so beneficial, women should be more conscious of consumption of vitamin D3!

The overall survival from some forms of ovarian cancer has not changed a great deal in the past 20 -40 years. Improvements in surgery and newer chemotherapy regimens may allow a longer period between diagnosis and death. For women diagnosed in Stage III, especially with advanced years at diagnosis, the recurrence of the cancer and death likely approach 100 percent. The life of an ovarian cancer patient may be prolonged for years but at a terrible price. There is no barrier or cover that exists to contain the spread of ovarian cancer. The liver has a capsule and the bowel has an outer membrane. The survival percentages for ovarian cancer are likely taken from Stage I and early Stage II.

With constipation, bloating, abdominal pain, and fatigue, one has a good reason to see a doctor. When the tumor is large enough, pressure may be applied on the bladder, causing frequent urination. Tumor pressure on the rectum can produce bowel symptoms of both constipation and diarrhea.

No other organ has as many different kinds of tumors as the ovary nor produces tumors as large. The record for the largest ovarian tumor is over 200 pounds. Epithelial cancers as ovarian cancer, are the most common, which are derived from the surface of epithelial cells of the ovary.

The most common route ovarian cancer takes is directly into the abdomen due to the sloughing off of the tumor cells from the outer surface of the ovary. The cancer cells block lymphatic channels and blood vessels. This causes production of ascites, the accumulation of fluid in the abdomen that needs to be drained off. The fluid is drained by inserting a catheter into the abdomen under CT or ultrasound guidance, known as paracentesis. Several liters of fluid can accumulate and become most uncomfortable for the patient. The fluid is composed of water, proteins, electrolytes, and amino acids. This accumulation is a drain on the patient's nutritional status and contributes to fatigue, weakness and loss of weight.

The CT scan (computerized axial tomography or CAT) and PET (Position Emission Tomography) are used to evaluate ovarian cancer. These tests show the body internal images as well as structural changes with great visibility. The two tests are identical except a radioactive sugar is injected intravenously prior to the PET scan. Cancer cells consume sugar and cancer nodules show up as lighted areas, whereas benign cells do not. Apparently, cancer tumors are devoid of sugar. Cancer cells consume sugar and the radioactive sugar used in the PET scan replenishes this lost sugar in tumors, consequently this area lights up like a "Christmas tree."

The term Stage is used to classify the degree of ovarian cancer from I to IV. Stage identifies the location indicating the degree of spread of the cancer. Ovarian cancer detected in Stage 1, generally has a good outcome. Only about 15-20 percent of ovarian cancers are detected in this early stage.

Generally, surgery is recommended when diagnosed with ovarian cancer. Cytoreductive surgery is the term used to describe this surgery. The term debulking, is also used. Debulking is not an inviting term although it is very descriptive of what really takes place. Depending on the Stage of the ovarian cancer, the following may be removed: uterus, fallopian tubes, ovaries, part of the omentum and lymph nodes. The omentum is the fat pad hanging down from the stomach. This is the area holding the liquid when referring to bloating. More extensive surgery (some times much more extensive) may be necessary as well.

The majority of ovarian cancer patients will respond to the first treatments of chemo. The first treatments of chemo will generally consist of carboplatinum (patented in 1972 and approved for medical use in 1989) and paclitaxel (Taxol). In December 1992, the FDA approved Taxol for treatment of ovarian cancer. Taxol was initially derived from the Pacific yew tree (Taxus brevifolia) in the 1960s and is now synthetically produced by a pharmaceutical company.

Both of these drugs have been used for about 30 years, so their use would not be innovative. Chemotherapy does not save most women with advanced ovarian cancer from recurrence and death. Chemo might be considered palliative for ovarian cancer since it extends life without eradicating the disease. It may keep the cancer at bay without eliminating it and extend life. Most women would choose chemo treatments over the alternative.

At some point the chemotherapy may stop working as efficiently as earlier in the treatment. It is speculation, but chemo may reduce the weaker cancer cells in the early treatments before they have had time to mutate repeatedly. The mutations may be more difficult to control. With time, the tumor metastasizes to the liver, breast, bowel, brain, lung or bone. A woman faces lethal metastases or treatments with side effects worse than those produced by the disease.

Chapter 3

OVARIAN CANCER, THE DEADLY INVADER

> Many things will work again, if unplugged for a while,
> including people.
>
> ----unknown

When studying ovarian cancer cells and the environment from which they originate, the unanswered question remains, how long does it take for normal cells to become malignant? The ovary is the only organ in the body with functioning cells facing the interior of the abdomen. Prior to the formation of a tumor, malignant cells become detached and are free to move. The detached ovarian cancer cells become attached or implanted on the surface of the liver, bowel, and elsewhere. This process is complicated and poorly understood. It is the presence of these nodules, especially around the bowel, that confers the discomfort alerting the patient that something is not quite right. Bloating, cramping. constipation, and abdominal pain are typical. Often, these are the symptoms of a small bowel obstruction.

The Pap smear is a welcome test. The Pap smear test is positive before the cervical malignant cells become invasive. The typical treatment is conducted in the office with a loop electrosurgical excision procedure (LEEP). This procedure allows the removal of the abnormality under microscopic guidance without injury do the uterus. Subsequent pregnancies are possible.

Ovarian cancer does not have such a test. Except in rare occasions, ovarian cancer patients lose the future possibility of pregnancy. Even if a woman has an annual exam which includes a pelvic exam, the Pap smear test, pelvic ultrasound and the CA- 125 (cancer antigen) blood test; ovarian cancer might be undetected. A routine annual pelvic examination may detect ovarian cancer in 1 of 10,000 cases. Over ninety-five percent of ovarian cancers are epithelial (covering) origin. There is no accurate diagnostic test for these tumors.

The long-term dream of mankind is that a vaccine will be developed to end the curse of cancer, as has been done in so many diseases of the past. Currently, the amount of cancer research is enormous, and is conducted by so many differing specialties. Articles are published but they may remain unrecognized by specialists that must move the information to the clinical level. The articles prepared for publication are deliberately written in such an obscure (technical) language as to discourage many readers. This is often interpreted as sophistication of the researcher attempting to impress peers. In many cases, it becomes a requirement in order to get a paper past reviewers before publication! As has, and will be pointed out, there has not been great breakthroughs in the treatment of ovarian cancer! The idea should be to push back the forest. Too often, research is little more than "copycat". When research is widespread over a 50-year period, and a half trillion dollars expended on research, results should be forthcoming. This certainly has not been the case with ovarian cancer.

The CA-125 (cancer antigen) blood test is a high molecular weight protein that may become elevated in patients with ovarian cancer. It is not 100 percent reliable, as some ovarian cancers are missed and some patients may have an elevated CA- 125 blood test and not have ovarian cancer. The test is best used in conjunction with imaging tests as CT scans and PET scans along with a biopsy. Some in the medical field tend to poor mouth the CA-125 blood test because it is not 100 percent perfect, but it is the only blood test they have for this cancer at this time.

The CA-125 blood test is used to monitor ovarian cancer treatment. As the treatment progresses, the CA-125 levels may drop off precipitously, if the treatment is working in a positive manner. If the CA-125 continues to rise, it can be a warning the drug(s) are not effective and the treatment needs to be terminated.

The CA-125 blood test has been noted elevated in 80 percent of patients with cirrhosis of the liver and nearly 50 percent of patients with pancreatic cancer. CA-125 levels may be as high as over 10,000. The CA-125 test is basically a test for inflammation and may test positive for gall bladder and urinary tract infections. It has been noted elevated in young women with endometriosis and benign fibroid tumors of the uterus. Roughly 20 percent of patients with ovarian cancer have a normal CA-125 reading. The CA-125 blood test has been used for over 30 years.

Two additional blood tests are available but both have an unacceptably low specificity rate. Neither has received universal acceptance. The first is OVA 1. It contains a number of compounds along with the CA-125 protein. The second is OvaSure. It contains the CA-125 protein along with other compounds as well. It would appear the development of a valid test would attract grant money to solve a serious problem of non-detection of ovarian cancer.

A sophisticated piece of equipment, called the microarray analyzer, may be promising in the early detection of ovarian cancer in the future. It measures the expression levels, that is, levels at which genes are activated in the human genome. Differences in expression patterns in cancer versus normal tissue from which cancer cells may arise might be identified. There are an estimated 20,000-25,000 genes in a human cell. It will be a day's work to be sure! Looks like an expensive piece of equipment with a lot of "mays" and "might", with no results.

In ovarian cancer surgery there is a mass in the ovary, tumor nodules on the surface of the bowel and omentum, the fat pad that hangs down from the stomach. Dissection of the cancer prior to its removal can be perilously close to such structures as the spleen, pancreas, kidney, and liver. The most common finding in patients with cancer of the ovary is a mass in the pelvis. Surgical procedures for cancer of the ovary are becoming more extensive with each passing year. It is questionable if the extended surgery is bringing the patient closer to a cure. It likely contributes to extending the life of the patient longer between diagnosis and death. Recovery from such extensive cancer must be the most tragic experience a woman must endure. The time of recovery might compare to an eternity and the pain endured unequaled.

There is an ongoing healthy debate regarding the use of preoperative chemotherapy to shrink the tumors and lessen the extent of the surgery. It may be just as well that there is no surgery at all in many cases of extensive invasion. Putting a woman through such a barbaric procedure with the weeks and months of pain to recover (partially), should be evaluated and well understood. Surgeons perform surgery! If there is no surgery, how much time will be lost?

Without surgery, chemotherapy can be initiated earlier. Cells divide and produce new daughter cells. Cancer cells divide more rapidly than normal cells. Cancer daughter cells divide before they have reached maturity. Chemotherapy slows down cell division. Note the term "slows down". Fortunately, cancer cells are far more sensitive than normal cells. Chemotherapy takes the good and the bad!

Some of the chemotherapy drugs currently given to patients with cancer of the ovary are listed below:

Carboplatinum (Carboplatin)
Paclitxel (Taxol)
Bevacizuab (Avastin)
Pegylated Liposomal Doxorubicin (Doxil)
Topotecn (Hycamtin)
Gemcitabine (Gemzar)
PARP inhibitiors (e.g. Olaparib)
Dicetaxek (Taxotere)
Etoposide (VP-16)
Xeloda (Capecitabine)
Arimidex (Anastrozole)
Tamoxifen (Nolvadex)

Taxol and Carboplatinum are the two drugs generally given during the early treatment for ovarian cancer. To deliver the drugs intravenously, a chest port in installed. This device is a small round plastic receptacle with a silicone rubber catheter attached. The port is placed just beneath the skin. The catheter is within a large vein near the heart. When the infusion needle is placed through the skin into the port, there is immediate access to the venous system.

Carboplatinum is excreted by the kidney rather than the liver. Serous kidney toxicity may result if the dose is not properly calculated. Kidney injury is often a common result of chemotherapy. **Neuropathy**, a numbness and tingling on the bottom of the feet is one of the common reactions to Carboplatinum. Gabapentin (**Neurontin**) is used to combat the neuropathy. Vitamin B6 sometimes relieves these symptoms as well. Oddly as it may seem, the cancer doctors were of little help in warning of these effects or recommending medications that would be helpful.

Both Carboplatinum and Taxol will cause hair loss, nausea, and bone marrow toxicity. This may result in a decrease in white blood cell count, red blood cell count, and platelet count, to dangerously low levels. If the white blood cell count drops low enough, in may cause a dangerous blood infection called *septicemia*.

Bevacizumab, or Avastin, is a vascular disruptive agent that interferes with blood vessel production. Avastin is not chemotherapy; it is a monoclonal antibody. It inhibits vascular endothelial growth factor (VEGF). The endothelium is the layer of cells that line blood vessels. Blocking the cancer's ability to make new blood vessels, Avastin can cause the tumor to shrink and can also reduce accumulation of fluid in the abdomen and chest.

Avastin has dangerous side effects. Excretion of protein in the urine is often experienced indicating injury to the kidney. Nosebleeds and changes in blood pressure are also reaction factors. The most serious complication with Avastin is bowel perforation. On occasion the tumor nodules on top of the bowel could dissolve so rapidly that an opening occurs in either the small or large intestine. Perforation of the bowel necessitates immediate surgery which may require a colostomy. Fortunately, the latter does not occur with any frequency.

Gemzar and Doxil are drugs used for recurrences of cancer, either by themselves or in combination with another drug. With all treatments of cancer, it must be restated that drugs are poisons and they have dangerous side effects. The dose and the interval between treatments depend entirely upon the ability of the body to withstand the repetitive poisoning. Age, physical condition, and weight of the patient certainly are parameters that must be taken into consideration.

A new group of drugs for treating ovarian cancer called PARP appear to offer great promise. These drugs inhibit the enzyme poly ADP ribose polymerase (PARP). This is an enzyme necessary in DNA repair. Standard chemotherapy drugs are poisons and insinuate themselves into the cell cycle at various stages of mitosis, or cell replication and division. The PARP inhibitor drugs alter the way DNA is repaired. This is a most complicated process.

Single strand breaks in DNA occur thousands of times daily in every cell. These breaks are repaired by the PARP enzyme by a method called base excision repair. PARP inhibitor drugs prevent the repair of single strand breaks in DNA. Single strand breaks that are not repaired become double strand breaks. These breaks are repaired by a process called homologous recombination. This is what the BRCA gene does. BRCA is a tumor suppressor gene. When double strand breaks cannot be repaired because of a mutation on the BRCA tumor suppressor gene, the cancer cell dies. Chemotherapy drugs may damage cancer cells without killing them. PARP inhibitors quicken cancer cell death. Chemotherapy drugs kill normal cells along with the cancer cells. PARP inhibitors do not kill normal cells.

PARP inhibitor drugs are: olaparib, iniparib, and veliparib. The oral medication olaparib (Lynparza) is available with a prescription. This drug is administered only under strict guidelines; there must be a deleterious mutation on one of the BRCA genes and there must be failure of three prior regimens of chemotherapy. Two percent of patients taking PARP inhibitors will develop acute myeloid leukemia or myelodysplastic syndrome (damage to blood-forming cells in the bone marrow). Almost all of these patients die of these complications.

Only 15 percent of ovarian cancer patients have a deleterious mutation on one of the BRCA genes. Myriad Genetic Laboratories has developed a homologous recombination deficiency (HRD) test which may be positive in up to 30 percent of patients who do not have a deleterious mutation on the BRCA gene. Such patients who test positive for HRD will be candidates for the PARP inhibitor drugs.

Ovarian cancer has a high recurrence rate. When imagining studies indicate widespread ovarian cancer, surgery is not an option and chemotherapy becomes the option of choice.

This discussion is an introduction to ovarian cancer. There are no early tests to alert the potential patient of ovarian cancer. The formation of cancer cells is extremely complex and poorly understood. The bottom line is that ovarian cancer formation and treatment is perhaps among the greatest challenges without solution in the field of medicine.

Chapter 4

THE NUTS AND BOLTS OF OVARIAN CANCER

Commitment is an act, not a word.

Anguish and devotion are two traits that any cancer victim lives with daily, some days are considerably worse than others. It is extremely difficult to fully realize that one's body has betrayed your life, your future, and how you will be spending your time for the foreseeable future. Now you must "live' with the frightful protocols of contemporary medicine and the people responsible for directing the course of your attempt to survive. Ovarian cancer in an incurable disease for most women diagnosed with this dreaded disease in the later stages. To date medical research has failed to find a cure for ovarian cancer and the recourse is the ineffective and injurious medical responses, that inflict great suffering and disappointment to the thousands of women so afflicted.

Patients, their loved ones, and the caregivers, deal with the disabling and frightful circumstances, with each turn of events, during the treatment process. The cry of all involved is that there must be something done to improve the miserable inadequacies of current medical research, trials, acceptance, and cure of ovarian cancer. Cancer patients live with death and their destiny is grounded in widely sanctioned health-care protocols. The urgency for cures is begging for solutions.

When a woman is first diagnosed with ovarian cancer, it has to be the worst lifetime curse she will ever experience. She may not fully realize the significance of this catastrophic diagnosis at the time. It may require extensive time before it fully sinks in. It is a time when those closest and most concerned will be grasping for words and actions to comfort the afflicted person. For far too many, it is a death sentence! How long will it be before a prevention of this cursed affliction will be resolved? For most, there is no cure, the treatments may be keeping patients alive longer with untold suffering.

Ovarian cancer remains the silent killer because, for most women, it is not diagnosed until Stage III or IV. The cancer is not discovered before it has spread to distant areas of the body. Only about 20 percent or less of ovarian cancers are discovered early in Stage I. For most, symptoms do not present themselves before the cancer has metastasized. Fluid buildup and constipation are the two main symptoms and that is because of the extensiveness of the cancer.

It is no secret that long-term survival rates show little improvement for over 50 years, in spite of information that is available to the contrary. The much-used quote, "People with ovarian cancer die of ovarian cancer," has not changed a great deal in relatively recent years. They just live longer with treatments.

It is not possible to conceive of the thoughts that women must experience who have been diagnosed with ovarian cancer. There is no way to understand what a stricken woman experiences between diagnosis and death or during initial and successive treatments. One of 78 women will be diagnosed with ovarian cancer in their lifetime, or about 1.3 percent. Also, death from ovarian cancer will occur in about 1 of 108 women. This does not seem like a large number if one is not afflicted. If you are the one diagnosed with ovarian cancer, this tragic diagnosis strikes frighteningly close to home. This is the deadliest disease of all gynecological cancers. There are few published personal accounts of women who have endured the curse of ovarian cancer. It is no longer necessary for women to remain silent about this silent killer! Cancer can strike anyone, anytime or anywhere. Cancer strikes, regardless of all of the factors of consideration as age, lifestyle, genetics, diet or any other perceived cause. An individual may help with some preventive factors but likely none are assured.

Women who are diagnosed with ovarian cancer have little free time, possibly the pain and suffering, coupled with fatigue and despair, prevent them from composing their story of the trials and tribulations they must endure daily. When a special-women dies, it is left to the survivor to construct her story. Too often, the survivor of this special person is too entangled in a fierce battle of grief, coping with his loss, to put the story together. And so, it goes untold!

Cancer of any kind brings devastating results. A diagnosis of cancer as ovarian cancer and others, brings just about the worst message that a person could phantom.

No one could be prepared for the horrific ordeals ahead for the women diagnosed with ovarian cancer. The feelings are multiple from possible severe depression to accepting the suffering more from the treatment than the disease. Current remedies have not been able to cure the disease; they often debilitate the victim until the afflicted person hardly recognizes herself. In the meantime, ovarian cancer survives as it has for centuries. New findings, the result of the research with unbelievable cost, have not achieved the desired outcomes of contemporary science. The women so condemned by the diagnosis of ovarian cancer, must endure the consequences of the incurable disease and accept the imminent fate! The success derived from gains in finding a cure for ovarian cancer have largely been arrived at by delaying the time of original diagnosis to the final death. A woman must weigh life-extending treatments against the fact that such treatments have the potential of destroying the pleasures of prolonged life. It ultimately must be realized that there simply is no cure for most cases of ovarian cancer. This is not the message emanating from the American Cancer Society or the nearest oncology center. The term palliative (medicine or medical care relieving pain without dealing with the cause of the condition) is out there for those who don't have the stomach for the suffering ahead with treatments. It is for those who can revert to letting events occur without interruption! It may be said that the term "palliative" is actually a description of existing ovarian care treatment except it comes with pain and discomfort or worse.

If a woman diagnosed with an incurable ovarian cancer should ask the question, why should I place myself in such a situation of suffering through all of the treatments, knowing that in the end I will die anyway? The answer lies in the realization that most women enjoying a happy, comfortable and satisfying life, will bargain for a few years, a few months, a few weeks, and then a few days!

Courageous women will address treatments for ovarian cancer as a chronic and treatable illness with elation and high hopes of a positive outcome. They have no other recourse. In more than 70 percent of cases whereby a woman is diagnosed with ovarian cancer, the cancer has already spread beyond the ovaries into the open space of the pelvic, omentum and elsewhere. Even with the best medical care, too many of these patients will suffer terminal results.

From infancy, we fear that something will take a life, as disease, an accident, a natural disaster, or whatever. No one knows the when, how, where or why one's life will end. Ovarian cancer that leads to a slow death at least gives the survivors some time to reconcile the outcome. It never lessons the maelstrom of grief, that awful feeling that is unshakable, the guilt of not doing enough, or saying the right things that you felt all along, but could not make yourself let it out. Food has no attraction, to the point that health of a surviving mate may be in danger. Grief is so awful; I have given consideration to the idea that it would be better if the grieving survivor in a loving relationship could just be given a pill.

Ovarian cancer is the silent killer; it sneaks up on a woman. It is insidious, meaning it is gradual; it may have been in progress for years or decades. No one fully knows how a normal cell changes to a cancerous cell or how long the time period might be. The way it is explained is, "A succession of genetic changes lead to the conversion of normal cells to cancer cells." That said, what does it mean? What is known is that it is undetectable, treacherous, slowly ensnaring the unsuspecting woman living in an active environment with her busy activities and coping with life. The ferocious treatment of the oncologist in treating a woman with advanced ovarian cancer, so ravages her body to the point that damage to a vital organ, such as the heart or kidney, actually is the cause of death. In a purely practical realization, this may actually be a better way to leave the world than the alternative wasting away, one day at a time, as the cancer ravages the flesh by consuming the proteins of the muscle and other tissue. It might be quicker and less painful for the patient. It says nothing for the cure of the cancer.

We live in a time where dramatic changes are occurring. The changes overwhelm us daily. Many things that we once used as the state of the art are now of the past. Advances have been made across the board in almost everything we could mention. This has not been the case for ovarian cancer. The statement was reportedly made at a medical conference that few ovarian cancer activists existed, because afflicted women didn't live long enough to become activists. Now a quarter century later, not much has changed in survival rates. Survival percentages are essentially meaningless. They are five-year survival estimates and the particular details of the survival are guarded and it is difficult to get usable data. It is an established fact that ovarian cancer kills more women than all other gynecologic cancers combined. It has been stated that if cancer is one of the most dreaded words in the English language, then for ovarian cancer patients, *ovarian* is the worst adjective there is to place before *cancer*.

In 2008, the overall median survival for ovarian cancer was given as 25 to 30 months. The most recent median survival that I have seen is 40 months. In the first case it meant that half of the women died in the first 25-35 months. In the second case, it means that half of the women died before 40 months. Then, it seems, progress has been made in widening the time of first diagnosis to the time of death. The reality is that remission requires follow-up treatment. When treatment stops, the patients suffer a relapse and die, leading a casual observer to assume that the diagnosis of late-stage ovarian cancer has the same connotation as a death sentence.

Ovarian cancer has warning signs. They too often are missed or dismissed. All that happens in a women's body from menstrual cycles, ovulation, birthing children, raising children and being the "master" of the household, possibly a job, and the many other activities in a woman's life, are considered "normal". Women experience many different and difficult reactions. They put up with these feelings and in a busy life style, ignore them for the most part. Two of the most repeated symptoms of ovarian cancer are constipation and bloating. Who has not experienced this feeling? Other symptoms may include fatigue, a reduced appetite, indigestion, recurrent back, abdominal or pelvic pain, urinary frequency, flatulence, irregular periods, spotting, shortness of breath, pain with intercourse or even incontinence. Should a woman have a medical examination when any of these symptoms occur? They would spend a great deal of time in the doctor's office. There is good reason that ovarian cancer is called the "silent killer." This is why people with ovarian cancer die of ovarian cancer!

It must be stated that some ovarian cancers may be misdiagnosed. With competent doctors and the support equipment available, this should not happen. It should also be stated that ovarian cancer is the great imposter. It masquerades as some of the most common symptoms in middle life and beyond.

The ovary is the olive shaped organ about the size of a pecan that contains all of the eggs in the complete course of a woman's fertility. When a female child is born, she will possess all of the eggs she will have in her lifetime. After reaching puberty, the two ovaries take turns in releasing eggs each 28 days. The eggs travel down the fallopian tubes where they may or may not be fertilized for the woman to become pregnant. The ovaries also produce hormones vital for a woman in the absence of which women take Estrogen and Progesterone. The ovaries have been difficult to study in the past and remain difficult to test and to treat because they are so deeply embedded within the body.

As early as 1809, both ovaries and the fallopian tubes were removed from a woman to relieve her of a cyst weighting more than twenty-two pounds. In 1805, a new substance was isolated from opium by Pharmacist Friedrich Serturner (1783-1841) that he named "morphium" after Morpheus, the god of dreams. In 1824 the German surgeon Karl Thiersch discovered cancer originating from epithelial cells. Epithelial cells originate from the tissue covering the lining of the ovary. Ether was available as early as 1846.

Ovarian cancer has been called Nature's revenge on the ambitious, childless woman. The current consensus is that continuous ovulation uninterrupted by pregnancy or oral contraceptive use, has the strongest correlation with ovarian cancer.

Mortality rates for ovarian cancer have not dropped dramatically over the past 50 years, as they have for other types of cancer. The length of time from diagnosis to death may have lengthened somewhat. The American Cancer Society does not release statistics like these but numbers as 70 percent of women diagnosed with Stage III and IV die within two years and the other 30 percent die within four or five years. The question, how long would such a woman live if she did nothing and went home and enjoyed every day she has left without the hassle of blood test after blood test and treatment after treatment that wrecks a woman's body? Is it true that ovarian cancer receives a small percentage of governmental research funding, research and little public attention?

Large pharmaceutical and Genetic companies have gained a series of patents that control new testing and drugs. The scarcity of product prices itself out of the market, when only one company controls production. A single shot to stimulate white blood cell count following a cancer treatment costs over $14,000, as just one example. Drugs proven effective for ovarian cancer are not available because of further governmental testing requirements, or simply lack of availability. The squeaky wheel gets the grease. Ovarian cancer may not be as important as other cancers when it comes to numbers. The money, research and potential outcomes goes for the volume. Deliverance of results is the only criteria on the table.

Chapter 5

THE CASE STUDY OF CELESTE

There is nothing harder than the softness of indifference.

----unknown

Celeste was in her 91st year when she was first diagnosed with ovarian cancer. This lady did not look nor act like a person of her age. She was extremely active, was at the YMCA gym five days a week, had a huge flower garden that she tended herself, was an active bridge player, attaining her Life Master status, an ex-pilot, and an avid reader. Each morning at breakfast she enjoyed mastering the crossword puzzle in the morning paper. She artistically formed each letter in caps with her expert engineering draftsmanship in ink. Her true relaxation and enjoyment included taking in a movie. She was retired as a career draftsman with several oil companies. Each morning, her first action was to collect flowers in bloom and arrange in vessels and place throughout the house, when in season. The local H.E.B. grocery store supplied flowers when local flowers were not available.

The earliest symptom that Celeste experienced was severe constipation. She was a private person and did not share her discomfort so I could not help her. She finally did relate to me that she was having a problem, and found relief with the help of the reliable twosome of prunes and prune juice.

The second symptom was bloating. Celeste was always so weight conscious and thought she was overeating so cut back on her food intake. The bloating persisted and worsened. I encouraged her to see a doctor but she refused. Finally, I made an appointment with the family doctor and she agreed to go but insisting there was nothing wrong with her. I might mention that Celeste was always very healthy, ate only healthy foods, was on no medication, and intended to make it to the age of 100. She did not drink coffee or tea. She was and looked the part of a person of excellent health.

On June 14, 2019 we were able to see a doctor for the first visit. She was x-rayed and a CT scan was scheduled for June 18. On June 20 the results of the CT scan were reviewed. An enlarged right ovary measuring 3.3 cm, was discovered on the CT scan. A large amount of ascitic fluid with probable omental metastasis was noted in the abdomen. The buildup of fluid occurred in the space surrounding the organs of the abdomen, called the omentum. Findings were suspicious for malignancy, possibly ovarian origin. The tissue of the omentum indicated a dense massive growth. When Celeste returned from the doctor's visit she announced, "I have some bad news!" This was the only time I did not accompany her on any of the multiple times we were in medical offices.

On June 20, a biopsy of the lower left side of the stomach was accomplished. At the same time the fluid (Paracentesis) was drained from the omentum. Over 100 ounces of fluid was removed and examined. Great comfort was achieved as a result of the drainage, but the fluid buildup was recurring due to the metastasizing cancer cells.

On June 26 we again met with the doctor to review the results of the biopsy. The ovarian malignancy was confirmed and identified as Papillary Serous Carcinoma, a highly malignant form of endometrial adenocarcinoma. This cancer is very similar to Uterine Serous Carcinoma (USC). It is clinically aggressive and a morphological distinct variant. It spreads more quickly than other more common forms of endometrial cancer. It began in the lining of the uterus (endometrium). It is a type II cancer, immune to hormone treatment.

The term "palliative" was used for the first time. The dictionary definition: "relieving pain or alleviating a problem without dealing with the underlying cause." This was also the last time the term was used as Celeste had no other intention than to attack the cancer as vigorously as humanly possible. She never had a view other than that the battle would be won.

Now it was time to move into the treatment phase. On June 28, we met with a cancer doctor for the first time. The doctor outlined the medical procedure for ovarian cancer; surgery and chemo therapy.

On July 10, we met with the surgeon, who also heads up all of the cancer treatments. The proposal was a series of six chemo treatments before surgery. The cancer was confirmed in Stage III. About 60 percent of ovarian cancer is diagnosed in Stage III. Only 15 to 20 percent is diagnosed in Stage I. No one in the medical arena will admit it, but I am confident that this cancer, Uterine Papillary Serous Carcinoma, is 100 percent fatal, particularly when an older person is involved when in Stage III or IV. The period between diagnosis and death may be extended due to treatment. But that is not a certainty. The statistics used by the American Cancer Association are estimates and they do not release survival rates on this particular cancer by age group and stage of diagnosis. I should add that Celeste was in top physical condition, having been involved in regular gymnasium activities for over 30 years. She continued gym activity during the time of her cancer treatments. In fact, she gave up none of her regular activities.

One statistic that is real is that ovarian cancer strikes one woman in 78 or about 1.3 percent of all women. As a comparison, one in nine will contract prostate cancer. Ovarian cancer takes on a far more realistic statistic when it strikes home. Celeste never showed any outward sign of cancer and never commented on "why" she was the one struck with cancer. She was extremely healthy and her life was built around healthy activities. She did all she could to live a healthy life full of activity and interests.

For ovarian cancer there is a blood test tumor marker known as CA-125, a cancer antigen. The "normal" range is 0-30. Celeste's number was 293.8.

On July 15, Celeste had a Power Port implanted in her upper right chest in proximity to a vein leading directly into the heart. The port is about the size of a quarter with a hole connected to a catheter to transmit the fluid chemo medication and other accompanying fluids into a large blood vein leading directly into the heart.

On July 17, we met with the local cancer doctor who outlined the plan of implementation of the chemo treatments. Only one chemical, Paclitaxel (Taxol), was to be administered during the first treatment to evaluate the patient's reaction to the chemical. Blood work was to be accomplished ten days following each chemo treatment. The CA-125 (cancer antigen) blood marker for ovarian cancer, as well as red and white blood cell count, was to be closely monitored. If Celeste is able to handle the first chemical, the second chemical would be added for the second treatment, three weeks later.

Next, we had a most important meeting with the financial officer to review potential charges. Celeste had both Medicare and Tri-Care and was assured that costs for the chemo therapy would be covered at no cost to her. The cost was estimated to be $120,000.

On July 19, Celeste had a dental hygiene appointment. It was discovered that she had a nerve reaction on the last lower molar on the left side. The dentist x-rayed the area and discovered that her jaw bone had lost bone density. His recommendation was to extract the tooth as early as possible in light of her Stage III ovarian cancer. Bone density and ovarian cancer are two different and separate entities and I do not know if there was any connection.

The tooth was extracted on July 22. The tooth was well anchored and fragmented when extracted. X-ray confirmed all parts of the tooth were removed. Although, a tooth fragment surfaced weeks later.

On July 23, we were at the hospital to have the fluid removed from Celeste's abdomen for the second time. It was preceded with a blood sample as always. An ultra sound is used to evaluate the fluid and the best location for entry for the drainage tube. The first drainage was on June 22, one month earlier. About three quarts of fluid was removed and needless to say, a great deal of comfort was realized. Celeste was now ready for a good meal and a rest.

Chapter 6

THE CHEMO TREATMENTS

There is only one thing worse than camping, and that is camping with other people.

----unknown

On August 1, the first chemo treatment was administered. We arrived for the 9:00 a. m. appointment and were met by the wonderful nurse supervising the Fusion area where the chemo treatments are given. She has 24 years of experience giving chemo treatments. She has a most pleasing personality with a positive outlook. All of the people we encountered have been simply wonderful.

Celeste was an upbeat cooperative trooper, ready to get on with the treatment. Throughout the entire ordeal, she never once showed any fear or doubt that the treatments would overcome her cancer.

Before chemo chemicals are administered, several other fluids are injected for infection, steroids, Benadryl, and nausea medication. All of which are important for the sake of the safety and well-being of the patient. Finally, around noon the first chemo chemical was injected, one drop at a time. It would be another three hours before the treatment was completed.

The Benadryl was highly effective and allowed Celeste to sleep or dose much of the time she was in the treatment chair. The nausea medication likewise was effective as she never experienced nausea. She had no infections and the steroids provided an energy boost to get her back home following treatment. It must be stated that one of the most critical functions involving cancer treatments has to do with the person preparing the solutions for injections. The different fluids must be prepared with precision. The cancer treatment chemical must be meticulously prepared considering height, weight, health concerns and age.

On August 2, we were back at the hospital to have the fluid drained from Celeste's abdomen for the third time. It had been only 10 days since fluid was drained previously. This permitted a monitoring of the fluid accumulation following the chemo treatment. Seven pounds of fluid was drained off.

The first noticeable reaction to the chemo treatment was pain in Celeste's legs and a burning sensation on the bottom of her feet. A soothing over-the-counter cream, Aspercreme, containing Lidocaine HCl at 4 percent strength, was used with some relief on her feet. This is nerve damage called **neuropathy**. She also uses a cream containing Lidocaine and Prilocaine, both 2.5 percent strength, to lubricate the port for chemo treatments.

Although Celeste was adamant about continuing her workout regime, she admitted her energy level was low. The steroids were helpful but the toll of the chemo surfaced. She did go to the Association pool in the housing area on August 6, but admitted she did not have energy to exercise intently as was her usual conduct in the pool.

Celeste was pleased to announce on August 6 that the intense pain in her legs had subsided after several days following the chemo treatment. She took Tylenol, 3,000 mgs per day for relief. The feeling of a burning sensation in her feet (**neuropathy**) continues. This is nerve damage from the chemo treatment, so the chemical in the chemo has reached the extremities. Trips to the local pool in the evening allow for physical exercise as well as a soothing environment for the bottom of her feet.

On August 9, Celeste had a blood sample taken as a follow-up to the first chemo treatment. Celeste looked thin and has lost weight in her buttocks and thighs as well as the usual places. She appears to have lost muscle.

On August 12 we visited the American Cancer Society office and picked out a wig.

August 13, Celeste's appetite picked up. She has lost 15 pounds due to a lack of appetite. It **was time to** add some weight before the next chemo treatment on August 22.

On August 15, Celeste shampooed her hair, while combing the wet hair, she noticed that hair accumulated on the brush. She lost a hand full. It was the first hair loss from the August 1 treatment, 14 days later. Hair loss is called "*Alopecia*"! Paclitaxel (Taxol) was the chemical administered at a dose rate of 290 mg/meter square. This is a hefty dose for a 91-year-old woman weighing 123 pounds. Celeste appeared to have handled it as best she could.

On August 16, the blood sample drawn on August 9 was reviewed. The white blood cell count had fallen from 6.6 to 4.6 following the first chemo treatment. *Neutropenia* is the term used for low levels of white blood cells. The HCT, Hemato crit, percent of red blood cells, had fallen from 37.7 to 36.7. The range for HCT is 37-47. She was border-line on the red blood cell count before start of the chemo treatments.

On August 17, Celeste is free of pain except for the burning sensation on the bottom of her feet. This nerve damage is uncomfortable and continues.

August 22, the second chemo treatment is administered with no noticeable consequences. The treatment included two chemicals; *Carboplatin* (285 mg.m2) and *Paclitaxel* (285 mg/m2).

On August 23, Celeste received a shot in the stomach of *Erythropoietin (EPO)* to boost the body's bone marrow to produce more white blood cells. She experienced pain in the hips and knees, as a result of the shot. These are the large bones and it indicates the EPO was working. She has been taking Tylenol to dull the pain. The burning sensation due to nerve damage, neuropathy, continues unabated and it looks to be a permanent ailment.

On August 30, blood was drawn following the second chemo treatment. Celeste went to the local pool with an upbeat attitude. She weighs 123, 5 pounds below her ideal weight. She has experienced some problems with balance. She did go to the YMCA for exercise classes four days this week and missed one day due to a doctor appointment.

On August 31, Celeste was up early, changed the bed linen, put fresh sheets on the bed, set up breakfast and then was outside to harvest any flowers ready for the vases. After breakfast, she had a day's work on her mind. First, she had to finish the Saturday crossword Puzzle, the hardest of the week. Each morning, Celeste finished the newspaper crossword puzzle to perfection with her engineering drawing lettering.

Celeste stretched this day as far as she had energy. She went to the library for a resupply of books. She always gets four with movies thrown in. Then she headed to the nursery to pick up potted flowering plants to replace those that did not withstand the heat.

On September 13, we had a review of the blood sample taken following the second chemo treatment. The CA-125 cancer marker had dropped from 293 to 116. This was a hopeful outcome.

Celeste feels good; she is active, goes to the gym in the therapeutic pool, swims in the local pool, has a good appetite and sleeps well. She is losing her hair; she has pain in her large bones (bone marrow) from the shot to stimulate white blood cells.

On September 16, Celeste received her third chemo treatment. Both chemicals were delivered and everything went well.

On September 17 we had the after-chemo treatment shot to boost white blood cells. This is the shot that causes pain in the large bones a few days after administering the shot and it lasts for about five days.

On September 20, a CT scan was accomplished. No food or water for four hours prior to the appointment. As usual, blood was drawn prior to the scan. Celeste had to drink two large containers of a chalky solution over a period of two hours. Then an intravenous port was installed in her arm to permit a drip solution for the CT scan. After three hours, Celeste was hungry and ready for a nap.

On September 23, blood was drawn for a complete blood analysis. On September 25, with the information of the CT scan and most recent blood sample, the surgeon determined that Celeste would receive three more chemo treatments, three weeks apart, before surgery. The CA-125 ovarian cancer marker was further reduced to 51.8 after the third chemo treatment. The CT scan indicated that there had been no reduction in the size of the enlarged ovary on the right side. The ovary is greatly swollen and more than twice the size of a normal ovary.

It must be remembered that the cancer was stage three when first diagnosed. The cancer cells had metastasized from the origination in the ovarian area to the large cavity below the rib cage called the omentum. The fluid from the metastasized cancer cells was responsible for the fluid buildup. The chemo treatments have the mission of stopping cancer cells from dividing and multiplying. Judging from the CA-125 reading, this part of the treatment has been successful.

On September 26, Celeste picked up a $150 wig provided by the Community Cancer Association. She wore the wig to the YMCA for a gym workout on September 27 and her hair looked almost natural!

To date, Celeste continues to be active in the gym and water aerobics. She has been active with all of her activities. Continuing care of all of her indoor and outdoor plants and household chores as though nothing has happened. The morning crossword puzzle is completed in record time with engineering precision. Each Monday, she plays competitive bridge with her partner. Often, she brings home the top prize for the best bridge score.

On October 7, Celeste had her fourth chemo treatment. It was like the two previous treatments preceded with a blood draw. The session lasted five and a half hours. The Benadryl induces sleep helping to make the time pass faster. The blood test indicated the white blood cell count was down to 4.1, with the low reading on the chart being 4.4.

Celeste continues to do well. She has endured the chemo treatments with near her normal activities. Her energy level remains good and she accomplishes almost everything she desires.

On October 28, Celeste had her fifth chemo treatment. The CA-125 was 52.1. The most recent blood test indicated her white blood cell count dropped to 3.8 from 4.1. The red blood cell count dropped to 35.9 from 36.9. The chemo treatments are quite standard. Six solutions are prepared for each treatment, only after the patient arrives in the treatment area. The logic is that the treatment solutions are quite expensive and they are prepared when the scheduled patient arrives. Two solutions, one for short term and one for long term nausea control, an antibiotic solution, a Benadryl solution, a steroid solution and finally the chemo chemicals. The line of the portal for the treatment solutions is flushed with saline solution after addition of each solution. Over a liter of solution is injected with each treatment. Celeste has tolerated the chemo treatments very well and only the burning sensation on the bottom of her feet remains persistent. During the chemo treatment, she is able to make a bathroom stop as the dispensing stand is on wheels and follows her. Otherwise, she is confined to a reclining chair for the usual five plus hours when receiving the chemo treatments.

On October 29, the regular post chemo treatment shot was given to boost the white blood cell count.

The day following chemo is a high energy day as the steroid provides an energy boost. Days following the shot to boost white blood cell production are downers. The chemo treatment takes its toll on the overall system. Celeste is more unstable on her feet; has low energy and needs to rest more as the poison of the chemo chemicals reacts. She stubbornly goes to the gym during this time, spending more time in water aerobics. She is determined to maintain her strength as she feels that this will be important to recovery from surgery and to tolerate future chemo treatments. Overall, her appetite is good, she sleeps well, and her weight has nearly recovered to precancerous status. Week two and three following chemo treatments have been good weeks for energy, freedom of pain, and productive achievement. Her outlook remains highly positive.

On November 18, Celeste had the sixth chemo treatment and the last treatment scheduled prior to surgery. As a reward, she was allowed to ring the bell reserved for chemo patients who have completed their schedules.

On November 19 Celeste received her regular scheduled white blood cell booster shot.

On December 2, the normal blood sample following the November 18 chemo treatment was taken.

On December 5, Celeste had a PET scan. She was injected with a radioactive sugar substance an hour before entering the scanning chamber. This scan is to highlight "active" tumors as opposed to scar tissue. Cancer cells deplete glucose sugar in the tumor cells. The radioactive sugar that is injected, reaches the sugar depleted tumor cells and displays the tumor locations. The cancer tumor locations are identified as lighted from the radioactive sugar.

On December 11, Celeste met with the surgeon to review the cancer treatments to date and to discuss potential upcoming surgery. The latest PET scan and latest blood samples were reviewed. The surgeon announced that the ***cancer is gone***! The ovarian cancer marker, CA 125, dropped to a normal of 27. The PET scan, used to identify active tumors, showed only dead and scar tissue. There was no comment made about the enlarged ovary.

The statement, "the cancer is gone" was made by the surgeon in charge of cancer treatments, This may have been a prelude for what we were to encounter in the future from this doctor.

Surgery was scheduled for December 26. The surgeon stated that surgery will remove the dead and scar tissue and that the tissue would be biopsied. We never saw any results of any biopsy. It was also announced that a quarterly blood test would be used to monitor any revival of the cancer cells. Nothing would be done in the interim to prevent the cancer cells from returning. We never heard any comment on the status of the swollen ovary!

December 26. Robotic surgery was performed. The surgery involved four vertical incisions each about one-inch in length, all above the waistline. The surgical incisions were positioned such that Celeste was essentially pain-free the days immediately following surgery. Obviously, consideration is given to the various muscles, knowledge of the physiological functions permits incisions in areas that result in little or no pain following surgery. Celeste spent one night in the hospital. There was no discussion about removal of the enlarged ovary!

On the morning after her stay in the hospital, we walked around the corridors of the hospital and Celeste appeared to move without any tenderness from the surgery. When we got back to her room, we were informed that she would be discharged from the hospital. It is always good news when anyone is informed that they can leave a hospital. By early afternoon, we were on our way home. The message that the cancer was "gone" was first and foremost on our minds.

Chapter 7

HIGH HOPES GOING INTO 2020.

When holding an elephant by the hind leg and it wants to run, let it go!

----unknown

January 8. We met with the surgeon to get a reading on the treatment status following surgery. Based on the biopsy taken at surgery, the decision was made that two more chemo treatments would be scheduled, one on January 22 and the other on February 12.

January 22. 10:15. Blood sample, Chemo treatment (Infusion)

January 23, 10:40. EPO shot, white blood booster

February 12. 8:45 Infusion

February 13. 2:15. EPO shot

March 6. 11:00. Blood sample

March 11. 1:15. Cancer doctor

April 14. 1:30. Blood sample

April 17. 9:00. CT scan, No food.

April 22. 1:30 Blood sample. <u>CA-125 10.9</u>

This is precisely how chemo therapy should work. It took the cancer cells down to the "normal" (0-30) range. Chemo is never going to get them all and we knew going in that this was an aggressive cancer and it is sure to be back, although the doctor in charge of the case never mentioned anything. The surgeon doctor never relates any information and acts as if we do not have a right to know.

May 4. 6:30 Hospital. CT scan, no food.

June- No appointments.

July 9. 1O:00 Kidney Specialist.

The Cancer is back!

July 9. 11:15. Blood sample <u>CA-125 174.7</u>

The last infusion was on February 12. On April 22, the cancer antigen reading was 10.9 and on July 9 the cancer had recovered to a reading of 174.7. This was a six months period of no treatment. Had the treatment been started a month earlier, the cancer antigen value would obviously have been lower.

July 15. 9:00. CT scan. No food/drink.

July 22. 4:00. Cancer doctor

July 29. 9:45 Hospital CT scan
        2:45 Blood sample

August 3. 1:30. Hospital. Echogram

Note that seven months have passed since the last chemo treatment.

August 6. 9:00. First chemo treatment <u>(Infusion)</u> of second series.

August 20. 8:45. Blood sample. <u>Infusion</u>

September 3. 9:30. Blood sample. <u>Infusion</u>

September 17. 8:30. Blood sample. <u>Infusion</u> <u>CA-125 163.1</u>

Note: CA-125 dropped from 174.7.

October 1. 12:30. Blood sample. <u>Infusion</u>

October 15. 9:45. Blood sample. Infusion

October 21. 1:30 Blood sample.

October 26. 3:00 CT scan.

October 28. 1:30. Blood sample. <u>Infusion</u>.

November 12. 8:45. Blood sample. <u>Infusion.</u>

November 18. 11:00. Blood sample

November 25. 12:45. Blood sample, <u>Infusion</u>

December 9. 9:25. Blood sample,<u> Infusion</u>

December 23. 8:45. Blood sample, <u>Infusion</u>

January 6, 2021. 8:45. Blood sample, <u>Infusion</u> <u>CA-125 41.5</u>

January 13. 9:00. Surgeon doctor.

January 22. 9:45. CT Scan

February 24. 3:00 Surgeon doctor, Blood sample. <u>CA-125 29.6</u>

    The chemo therapy did what it was designed to do as it lowered the cancer antigen reading into the "normal" 0-30 reading once again. Now the important issue is to not let the cancer cells build to a high level before further treatment. The cancer cells need to be monitored and action needs to be taken before the cancer has a chance to recover extensively.

Celeste is able to condone the chemo treatments and leads a near normal life. As long as the chemo treatments can control the cancer cells, Celeste is managing. She has suffered kidney damage. We are awaiting the next challenge.

Chapter 8

A NEW CANCER TREATMENT

The old fella got the OK from his doctor to join an aerobics class. He jumped up and down, bent over, moved around, pulled and perspired. By the time hie got into his leotards, the class was over.

....unknown

Cancer has a way of returning with a vengeance, when not treated. Once the cancer cells get to the "normal" level of 0-30 on the CA-125 scale, they must be monitored closely. At the first sign of cancer rebuilding, chemo treatments must be reinstated. Any further delay allows the cancer cells to build rapidly and become more difficult to control. When something is working so well as the chemo treatments did on both occasions, there should be no hesitation to reestablish the chemo treatments, especially when they were so effective and the patient was able to tolerate the chemo treatments so well.

Note that there has been no cancer therapy since January 6, 2021.

March. No appointments

April. No appointments

May 24. 12:30 Urine sample, Blood Pressure 107/61,
No blood sample.

There have been no blood samples to indicate the cancer antigen reading. The doctor in charge of cancer treatments decided to forgo the chemo cancer treatments that were highly successful.

The statement that ovarian cancer remains a disease in search of a consensus, could never be more accurate!

The treatment selected by the doctor in charge of cancer was a generic drug called Mvasi. It is a biosimilar medical product that is almost an identical copy of an original medication manufactured by a different pharmaceutical company. The original medication is called Bevacizumab or Avastin. It is a vascular disruptive agent that interferes with blood vessel production.

Bevacizumab is classified as a "monoclonal antibody" and "anti-angiogenesis" drug that inhibits vascular endothelial growth factor (VEGF). The endothelium is the layer of cells lining blood vessels. In theory, Bevacizumab blocks the cancer's ability to make new blood vessels and cause the tumor to shrink as well as reduce the accumulation of fluid in the abdominal area. It is assumed the "biosimilar" drug Mvasi, would perform in a similar way.

The treatment was a combination of liposomal doxorubicin (Doxil) plus Mvasi. Doxil is to prevent cancer cells from dividing and growing, ideally to cause to shrink and die.

The Mvasi drug is to target cancer cells more precisely than chemotherapy. The greatest side effect of Mvasi is the increase in the incidence of excretion of protein in the urine.

A bowel perforation is a serious complication from the use of the Avastin-like Mvasi. The tumor nodules on top of the bowel may dissolve rapidly causing an opening in either the small or large intestines. This would necessitate an immediate surgery that might result in a colostomy.

On the surface, this treatment is recognized as a standard practice. Much has to do with the appropriate dose. The question, was there a protocol followed to ensure the dosage was correct? Was there any experience with these drugs previously? Were all involved certified to handle these chemicals?

The cancer is back!

June 14. 12:30 Blood sample, <u>Infusion</u> with new cancer chemicals.

First blood sample since February 24.

July 6. 10:30 Blood sample, <u>Infusion</u>

July 22. 12:30. Kidney Specialist.

July 27. 9:30 Blood sample, <u>Infusion</u>. CA-125 363.1

    The cancer antigen test was finally recorded and it had skyrocketed to 363.1 and the new "experimental" chemicals selected had absolutely no effect. The doctor had allowed the cancer antigen test to exceed all previous levels.

    After three disastrous treatments the doctor terminated the cancer treatment. Among other things, the chemical had further damaged Celeste's kidneys and it had no effect on lowering the cancer antigen reading.

    Following cancellation of the Mvasi, on July 27, two more months passed before there was any treatment. In all, seven months passed without an effective treatment. Mvasi is not a chemo and is classified as a "monoclonal antibody" an "anti-angiogenesis" drug.

August 16. 9:30. Blood sample. <u>The CA-125 was 571.1,</u> up from 363.1 on July 27.

August 23. 9:30. CT scan.

August 25. 3:20. Surgeon doctor appointment

On September 9, Celeste had an 8:00 appointment with Cardiology as she was having heart issues.

The next drug to be tried was Gemcitabine or Gemzar.

September 17. 2:45. Blood sample, first <u>infusion </u>of Gemzar.

Note the last infusion was on July 27.

September 24. 10:15. Blood sample. No CA-125 blood test.

September 29. 8:00. Echocardiogram

October 1. 10:45. Blood sample. No CA-125 blood test.

October 13. Cardiology and blood sample.

October 14-16. Celeste hospitalized due to potassium level spiking in her blood.

October 18. Blood sample. <u>CA-125 695</u>

October 19. 9:15. <u>Infusion</u>

October 27. 1:15. Blood sample, <u>Infusion</u>

November 1. 2:40. Cardiology.

November 4. 8:00. CT scan. No food or drink.

November 5. 11:00 Blood sample. <u>CA-125 729.5</u>

November 10. Surgeon doctor appointment

This was the meeting when this doctor decided that since the wrong chemicals for treatments for Celeste did not work, all treatments were to be terminated and Celeste was to be sent home to die.

The usual five minutes or less time was utilized. The doctor sat down on the stool and the first thing stated was since nothing seemed to be working, all treatments would be terminated and that Celeste would be turned over to Hospice (to die).

Those words of termination of treatments were devastating. Consider anyone in the same position. Here is a doctor condemning you to die because selection of chemicals for your treatment did not work. There was no obligation to not continue the chemo treatments. This was a decision made by this doctor alone. The words, "Ovarian cancer remains a disease in search of a consensus" could never be more-true!

The doctor was cold and heartless. It was shocking. Here the doctor was playing God, determining who would live and who would die. In my view, all because the doctor made the wrong decisions and poor choices.

It is a redundancy to say the chemo treatments worked. In both of the chemo series, the CA-125 was in the normal range when the treatments were completed. Here was a case of a 93-year-old lady tolerating the chemo treatments and doing well. This doctor put aside a treatment that has been doing its job for 30 years. A highly dependable treatment that proved itself to be effective on both occasions it was used, caused Celeste no nausea, and she was able to tolerate it and lead a near normal life.

It is my understanding that chemo can be given up to six times. Chemo was administered in two series with astounding success. There is no indication that the chemo would not have been successful a third time. Each series of treatments totaled about one year. Each successful treatment series adds about one year to survival. Celeste was a young 93.

Celeste undertook the cancer treatments because she wanted to live. She did everything she was asked to do for treatment of her cancer. She had complete trust in the doctor. Now she was told to go home and sign up for Hospice and wait! (And die)!

Celeste was not cancer-eaten. She was not so emaciated that she was in a wheel chair unable to hold her head up. Celeste looked like she was ready to go out dancing, picnicking in the park, take a cruise, or any of a number of activities. She had just returned from a week at South Padre Island where she frolicked in the water attacking the breakers. She loved to walk the beach bare-footed and feel the clean, fine sand under foot. The sea breeze was so stimulating to her. Yes, her body was full of cancer, but only because of the incompetence of the doctor. How bitter those awful words uttered to Celeste had to sound. This doctor had no difficulty with the wording and I am confident could utter them to anyone!

I seriously question the judgment of this doctor. I question her ethics as well. Here the doctor thought a decision had to be made to use different chemicals from the ones that worked. This is without rhyme or reason. This is where I question the judgement. It would have been so easy to continue the chemo therapy. Why wait five months before giving any treatments. There was not even interest in getting a CA-125 blood sample reading. If it was thought that cancer cells were getting the upper hand, how costly would it have been on everyone involved to continue the chemo treatments. It would appear to have been the "humane" decision to make.

A point I would like to make about the medical community in general, but which especially applies to this doctor. I see a tendency for doctors to look at the date of birth and generally apply it across the board. Celeste was in good physical condition and was far younger than her birth date when compared to others the same age. She loved life and she had so much to live for. She endured the chemo treatment to extend and enjoy life and now that was taken away from her.

Chapter 9

HIGH-GRADE SEROUS OVARIAN CARCINOMA

Surgeons must be very careful
When they take the knife!
Underneath their fine incisions
Stirs the Culprit—life!

Emily Dickinson

This is a common type of cancer accounting for about 75 percent of epithelial cancers. Many high-grade serous ovarian carcinomas (HGSOC) originate in the epithelium of fallopian tubes. High-grade serious carcinoma cells and tissue viewed under a microscope appear highly abnormal compared to healthy cells and tissue. High-grade carcinoma tumors are poorly differentiated, meaning they do not have a clear structure or pattern. Tumor cells originate abnormally and grow quickly. High-grade serous ovarian carcinomas are classified as Grade 3. "Serous" means that the tumor originated from the serous membrane in the epithelial layer in the abdominopelvic cavity.

This is an advanced stage carcinoma that generally spreads to the peritoneum (the lining of the organs of the pelvis and abdomen) first and leads to fluid buildup, called ascites, in the peritoneal cavity, resulting in bloating of the abdomen.

Serous adenocarcinoma or USC, is a rare subtype of endometrial cancer that is very aggressive, with high risk. Women diagnosed with this type of cancer should take care of matters that are highly important and enjoy each and every day. This cancer represents less than 10 percent of uterine cancers, and 80 percent of deaths from endometrial cancer.

Human cancers develop through a multi-step process that is extremely complex and poorly understood. In fact, so complex and sophisticated that "The war on cancer may never be won: Cure could be impossible because the disease is so highly evolved." (Lizzie Parry. http://www.daily mail. co.uk/health/article January 31, 2017)

Ovarian cancer is the third most commonly diagnosed cancer and the second leading cause of reproductive system death-related mortality in 2020. (Sung et. al, 2020)

Worldwide, 313,959 cases of ovarian cancer were diagnosed in 2020 and 207,252 died, or 72 percent. The five-year survival rate for ovarian cancer remains around 25-35 percent, and most of these were likely diagnosed in first or early second Stage. (Lee et al. 2018)

There is little question that ovarian cancer is a deadly gynecological cancer. The tumor microenvironment (TIME) plays a pivotal role in ovarian cancer development and the length of time of development of ovarian cancer is not known.

It has been stated earlier that Dr. Susan Love is credited with the statement that it takes 100 days for one cell to double. Most breast cancers have been present for 8 to 10 years by the time one can feel the smallest lumps. This says that cancer takes a long time to develop.

It is a common observation that when ovarian cancer gets going, it is very fast-moving.

The present concept continues to identify the location of the origination of ovarian cancer as the end of the fallopian tubes. Surgery to remove the tumor remains the most common treatment in the initiation of treatment for ovarian cancer. Celeste had a fibroid tumor removed when in her early thirties. The doctor performed a limited hysterectomy and left one ovary. Tragically, this is the ovary that was the source of her cancer.

The relationship of milk and ovarian cancer continues to be studied. The component in milk that appears to be the causative factor of milk is the simple six carbon sugar, galactose. An eight-ounce glass of milk contains 450 mg of free galactose and 10 g (10,000 mg) lactose. Lactose breaks down to one molecule of glucose and one molecule of galactose. Given equal value for glucose and galactose in lactose, one glass of milk contains 5,450 mg of galactose. One serving of hard cheese, about 28 g, contains 25 mg of galactose and no lactose.

Long-term consumption of milk may be more prevalent to chronic diseases like ovarian cancer with a long duration of development. Animal studies have shown that high dietary consumption of galactose causes ovarian toxicity.

A study in Sweden concluded that consumption of more than one glass of milk daily doubled the risk of serous ovarian cancer. (November issue of American Journal of Clinical Nutrition, 2004)

With ovarian cancer, there will often be a mass in the ovarian section and tumor nodules on the surface of the bowel and a deposit of tumor in the omentum, the fat pad that hangs down from the stomach. The bladder and rectum may have tumor tissue as swell. The interior or the entire abdominal cavity is at risk for tumor growth.

Surgery is generally suggested as the first ovarian cancer treatment. Many surgeries are so extensive a woman undergoing such surgery may wonder if there is going to be anything left after the surgery.

The first weeks following surgery must be an absolute miserable existence. Older women might be excused from such surgery.

The next phase is chemo therapy. In the previous chapters, chemotherapy is discussed. It is doable and it appears the only choice for most cancers.

When all treatments fail, tumors metastasize in the liver, breast, bowel, brain, lung, or bone.

In the later stages of ovarian cancer, carcinomatosis, the proliferation of tumors throughout the body, frequently causes ascites (fluid obstructing the diaphragm), bowel obstruction that may require a PEG (percutaneous endoscopic gastrostomy) tube to provide continuous drainage. Abdominal blockage may require a NG (nastogastric tube). Lymphedema is fluid retention in the lymphatic system. Kidney obstruction may require nephrostomy tubes or stents. Fistulas (abscesses), dyspnea (difficulty breathing) and malnutrition may be part of the problems to be experienced.

Chemotherapy might be considered palliative for ovarian cancer since it extends life without eradicating the disease. It may keep cancer at bay without eliminating it. Chemotherapy and other cancer treatments do not keep most women from recurrence and death from late-stage ovarian cancer.

Chapter 10

MILK AND OVARIAN CANCER

The less people know, the more stubbornly they know it.

.......unknown

Ovarian cancer is the second most common gynecologic cancer behind uterine (endometrial) cancer in the U.S. Ovarian cancer causes more deaths than any other cancer of the female reproductive system. The American Cancer Society estimates that over 22,000 women will be diagnosed with ovarian cancer and 12,810 will die in 2022 of ovarian cancer. In 2021, worldwide 313,959 cases of ovarian cancer were diagnosed and 207,252 died. The five-year survival rate for ovarian cancer remains around 25-35 percent. (Lee et al. 2018)

The lifetime chance of dying from ovarian cancer is about 1 in 108 women. About half of the women diagnosed with ovarian cancer will be 63 years old or older.

Milk has long been suspected as contributing to ovarian and breast cancer. There was a flurry of research around the turn of the century on this subject, but then, current research has almost disappeared in the further study of milk and dairy products as related to ovarian and breast cancers. The Dairy Promotion Council, better known as the American Dairy Association (ADA) has much political support. I have long jokingly referred to the ADA as the milk mafia. The ADA supported research of this nature would certainly be reviewed in such a way that there would be no conclusive correlation between milk or dairy products and cancer.

According to the United States Department of Agriculture (USDA), American milk consumption dropped from 275 pounds (32 gallons) per capita in 1975 to 149 pounds (17.3 gallons) in 2017, a 47 percent decrease. In 2020, milk consumption had further dropped to 141 pounds (16.4 gallons) per capita. In 2021 fluid milk consumption had decreased to 135 pounds (15.7 gallons) per capita.

The U.S. dumps millions of gallons of excess milk a year. In 2016, the American dairy industry dumped 43 million gallons of excess milk in fields, animal feed, or anaerobic (without oxygen) lagoons. The federal government purchases billions of dollars' worth of excess milk, which ends up stored as cheese. As of 2019, the USDA had 1.4 billion pounds of surplus cheese.

With the passage of the Agricultural Act of 2014, the dairy industry received $43 billion in 2016 and $36.3 billion in 2017. In 2018, 42 percent of revenue for the US dairy producers came from government support.

By 2006, small farms with fewer than 30 cows produced just over 1 percent of all dairy production.

Milk and milk by-products are leading contributors to the $1.3 trillion sickness industry. Milk and dairy products are linked to allergies, gas, constipation, obesity, cancer, heart disease, infectious diseases, and osteoporosis.

Several studies have concluded that drinking milk is more likely to cause than to prevent osteoporosis, the leaching of calcium from the bones due to the casein-protein in milk.

A cup of calcium-enriched orange juiced contains more calcium than a cup of fortified milk, 350 milligrams versus 302 milligrams. Bone mass stops after about age 35. Calcium from many food sources, plus calcium supplements, supplies sufficient calcium for maintenance of bone density.

Milk contains hormones and infectious diseases. Next to the human mouth, milk is the second most ideal medium for bacterial multiplication. Commercial dairy herds receive bovine growth hormone (BGH) injections to increase milk production. Bovine growth hormone is also known as bovine somatotropin. Somatotropin (bst) is naturally produced by cows. It is also known as a human growth hormone in its human form. It is a peptide hormone produced by the pituitary gland that stimulates growth, cell and reproduction. The age of puberty, and breast development are affected by these hormones.

The introduction of BGH and the extra hormones added to milk have contributed to the increase in the size of the average teenage human female breast and have decreased the age of menarche (ovulation) (Yoffe, Emily, "Got Osteoporosis? Maybe All That Milk You've been Drinking is to Blame," Slate Magazine, www.slate.com. 2 August 1999.) Children began ovulation when very young and it is not possible to state the earliest age of ovulation. We do have the story of the pregnant 10-year-old from Ohio who received much publicity about an Indiana abortion in July of 2022. How much of this early development can be attributed to hormones in cow's milk?

Milk cows also receive antibiotics. The United States Department of Agriculture (USDA) allows grocery store milk to contain 750,000 white blood cells per milliliter, based on bulk-tank somatic cell counts for Grade A milk producers (after milk is comingled from many sources.)

One 12-ounce glass of whole milk contains as much saturated fat as eight strips of bacon, 300 calories and 16 grams of fat. The ADA lobbied Congress to subsidize overproduction of milk. Milk, as a part of mandatory school lunch programs, followed. Many children and adults are lactose (the milk sugars in milk) intolerant.

In addition to fortified orange juice, soybean extract is used to produce soy milk. Unlike milk, soy does not contain the casein-protein in milk that results in calcium loss in bones leading to osteoporosis. The isoflavones found in soybeans can increase bone mineral content and bone density. (Soy has no hormones, antibiotics, no pus, etc.) (www.unitedsoybeanboard. com). Another soy isoflavone, genistein, stops cancer cells from growing when added to live cancer cells in laboratory test tubes.

Genistein, an isoflavone, was identified in 1928. Biotransformation of genistein by intestinal microbes is known to produce phytoestrogen equol. This phytoestrogen has potential anticancer activity. It is a nonsteroidal estrogen. Equol is of interest in many malignant diseases.

Genistein exists at relatively low concentration in the blood. Epidemiologic studies have demonstrated a significant difference in cancer prevalence based on dietary intake. Genistein has been shown to inhibit development of primary tumors in animal models. Genistein has been shown to be an antioxidant, a modulator of inflammation, and inhibitor of epigenetic changes.

Additionally, soybeans contain more protein by weight than beef, fish, or chicken, with no cholesterol and little saturated fat. Soy protein is the only "complete" vegetable protein. Humans require 20 basic amino acids which are derived from proteins, 11 of which can be produced by the human body. The remaining nine amino acids are called "essential" as they must be derived from outside the body from foods consumed. Soy protein provides all nine of these essential amino acids.

As an aside from this discussion, a word about the origination of the soybean plant. Soybeans first came to North America in the early 1800s, not as a food but as ballast aboard clipper ships. In 1904, George Washington Carver, the famous African-American chemist, son of a slave, whose owner was Moses Carver, discovered the high-protein value of soybeans as an animal feed. Henry Ford used soybeans to make plastic parts for many Ford cars, using 60 pounds of soybeans in every Ford by 1935. In 2855 B.C., Emperor Sheng-Nung of China named five sacred plants: soybeans, rice, wheat, barley and millet. (www.ncsoiy.org.) The soybean plant came from China.

A study from Harvard Medical School first reported in May of 2000 that nurses who consumed two or more glasses of milk daily had an increased ovarian cancer risk of 44 percent compared to women who rarely drank milk.

The Harvard Medical School study involved 80,326 married nurses living in 11 states. The study was initiated in 1976, and the nurses ranged in age from 30 to 55. Kathleen M. Fairfield, MD, and her co-authors reported on 16 years of dietary studies. There were 301 cases of ovarian cancer diagnosed during the 16 years and 174 ovarian cases were serous tumors (58 percent). The serous tumors are a rare subtype of endometrial ovarian cancer and are deadly. They are clinically aggressive, a morphological distinct variant which spreads more quickly than other more common forms of endometrial cancer. In this study, 58 percent of the ovarian cancer patients had the high-grade (deadly) serous tumors. Uterine serous carcinoma (USC), an aggressive variant of endometrial cancer, accounts for less than 10 percent of all endometrial cancers and 80 percent of endometrial cancer related deaths.

In the study, the nurses were getting 57 percent of their dietary lactose from low-fat or skim milk, 15 percent from whole milk, and 8 percent from yogurt. Cheese is low in lactose. Other studies have shown that low rates of milk consumption correlate well with low rates of ovarian cancer, especially serous tumors.

Milk has been identified as the dairy product with the strongest single positive association with ovarian cancer. In the November 2004 issue of the American Journal of Clinical Nutrition, participants who drank more than one eight-ounce glass of milk daily had twice the cancer risk as those who drank one eight-ounce glass of milk or less daily. Low fat or skim milk did not matter.

Neither the fat in milk nor the calcium content of milk increases the risk of ovarian cancer. Lactose, the milk sugar, appears to be the most likely culprit. An eight-ounce glass of cow's milk contains about 11 grams of lactose and about 450 milligrams of galactose. As a comparison, one serving of hard cheese (28 grams), contains 25 milligrams of galactose and no lactose. In the digestive process, the milk sugar, lactose, breaks down to form two six-carbon sugars, glucose and galactose. The milk sugar linked to cancer growth appears to be galactose. Lactose-free milk contains galactose. It is the casein-protein in milk that results in calcium loss in bones initiating osteoporosis. About 80 percent of cow's milk protein is casein. Human milk has a particularly low casein content. Calcium supplements may be a much safer route for women who are conscious of osteoporosis (and stop all consumption of milk and dairy products.)

A Swedish study reported that women who consumed two glasses of milk or more daily, had double the rate of ovarian cancer compared to women who drank only one glass of milk, or less, daily.

Ovaries may be prone to galactose toxicity owing to their high local concentration of the galactose-metabolizing enzyme, galactose1-phosphate uridyltransferase, as well as their high tissue-specific activity of the enzyme. (Xu et al. 1989, Larsson et al 2004).

Galactose is believed to be ootoxic or to induce high concentrations of gonadotropins (Cramer, 1989; Cramer et al. 1989).

Gonadotropins are two hormones, luteinizing hormone (LH) and follicle-stimulating hormone (FSH), which are produced by the pituitary gland. These hormones stimulate the ovaries to produce a follicle, which contains an egg (oocyte) and to release the egg from the ovary. With additional gonadotropins, there is a 30 percent increase in conceiving twins.

Lactose had a toxic effect on oocytes and prematurely raised gonadotropins in mouse/rat models. High lactose diets led to ovulatory disfunction.

Ovarian cancer begins at the end of the fallopian tubes. Ovarian cancer is a deadly gynecological cancer. The tumor immune microenvironment (time) plays a pivotal role in ovarian cancer development and the length of time of development of ovarian cancer is not known. As indicated earlier, it takes an average of 6.5 years for the cancer cells to move from the fallopian tubes to the ovaries.

Long-term consumption of milk may be more prevalent to chronic diseases like ovarian cancer with a long duration of development. Animal studies have shown that high dietary galactose causes ovarian toxicity.

The highest incidence of ovarian cancer occurs in Scandinavian countries where many dairy products are consumed, especially milk, and particularly, if they consumed more than one glass of milk daily. There are a number of studies implicating milk.

An interesting quote from Douglas Hanahan and Robert Weinberg, University of California, Hormone Research Institute, San Francisco, January 7, 2000. "After a quarter century of rapid advances, cancer research has generated a rich and complex body of knowledge, revealing cancer to be a disease involving dynamic changes in genome. Some would argue that the search for the origin and treatment of this disease will continue over the next quarter century in much the same manner as it has in the recent past, by adding further layers of complexity to scientific literature that is already complex, almost beyond measure." I might comment that the quarter century has nearly passed in 2022, and yes, there are many layers of complex scientific literature added, and I don't see that we are any closer to finding a cure for ovarian cancer now than we were a quarter century ago. I would very much like to be in error, but the statistics of the real determinator, death, supports my conjecture. Learning more about how a cell is changed into a malignant cell, is a start. How to stop the malignant cancer cell is the part of the battle that does not appear to be winnable.

Hanahan and Weinberg are active publishers of scientific papers and they have learned much about ovarian cancer. The next step is taking this library knowledge to the laboratory and to the cancer clinics. That is where the stumbling blocks are formidable. What they are explaining in their technical papers, is that ovarian cancer is extremely complex. There may never be a solution to this cancer and others as well. If a computer could be trained to outthink and find ways to outmaneuver ovarian cancer (and other cancers), a cure might be closer than it is today. In the meantime, more women will suffer and die from ovarian cancer, as well as other forms of cancer.

Ovarian cancer is not the only cancer affected by milk by any means.

Milk and other dairy products are the top source of saturated fat in the American diet, contributing to heart disease, type 2-diabetes, and Alzheimer's disease. Studies have also linked dairy to an increased risk of breast and prostate cancers.

Milk and other dairy products are the top sources of artery-clogging fat in the American diet. Milk products also contain cholesterol. Diets high in fat and cholesterol increase the risk of heart disease, which remains America's top killer. Cheese is especially dangerous. Typical cheeses are 70 percent fat.

Infants and children produce an enzyme (lactase) that breaks down lactose, the sugar found in breast and cow's milk. As they grow older, many lose this capacity and become lactose intolerant. About 95 percent of Asian Americans, 74 percent of Native Americans, 70 percent of African Americans, 53 percent Mexican Americans, and 15 percent of Caucasians are lactose intolerant. Symptoms include an upset stomach, diarrhea, and gas.

Studies of breast cancer implicate milk and dairy products as well. One study of nearly 10,000 women found that those who consume low-fat diets had a 23 percent lower risk for breast cancer recurrence. They also had a 17 percent lower risk of dying from the disease.

A 2017 study funded by the National Cancer Institute compared the diets of women diagnosed with breast cancer to those without breast cancer. They found that those who consumed the most American, cheddar, and cream cheeses had a 53 percent higher risk for breast cancer.

Among women previously diagnosed with breast cancer, those consuming one or more servings of high-fat dairy products (e.g., cheese, ice cream, whole milk) daily had a 49 percent higher breast cancer mortality, compared with those consuming less than one-half serving daily.

Research funded by the National Cancer Institute, the National Institutes of Health, and the World Cancer Research Fund, found that women who consumed 1/4 to 1/3 cup of cow's milk per day had a 30 percent increased chance for breast cancer compared to non-milk drinkers.

Regular consumption of dairy products has also been linked to prostate cancer. High intakes of dairy products including whole and low-fat milk increase the risk for prostate cancer, a study using meta-analyses that looked at 32 studies.

Another study revealed that men who consumed three or more servings of dairy products a day had a 141 percent higher risk of death due to prostate cancer compared to those who consumed less than one serving per day.

The research on galactose from the breakdown of the lactose sugar in milk is now a quarter century old and new research is lacking. The reasons may be obvious. The early studies have not been repeated and reconfirmed and the door is left open for skeptics. Sophisticated experimental designs have not proven within a 95percentile confidence limit assurance that a + b = c. Because it appears ovarian cancer and likely other cancers as well, take a long time to develop, perhaps a decade or more, women and men who have consumed milk over a long period of time, provide the perfect storm for cancer to develop. The older the population, the higher the risk.

Death is an abstract concept until its imminence slams into you. It was Voltaire, (1694-1778), who stated, "The art of medicine consists in amusing the patient while nature cures the disease." Voltaire was never introduced to ovarian cancer!

Celeste loved milk and considered it her dessert. She drank three glasses of milk daily most of her life. Ten years before she was diagnosed with ovarian cancer, she reduced her milk consumption to one glass per day. It is possible, that a decade ago the initiation of her ovarian cancer was well on its way. If it takes an average of 6.5 years for cancer cells to travel from fallopian tubes to the ovary, how long does it take to develop enough cancer cells to get the cancer machine rolling?

The high probability of death from uterine serous carcinoma, a rare subtype of endometrial cancer, (the type Celeste had) cannot be taken lightly. Chemo treatments are successful in lowering the CA-125 level, but the chemo treatments are not effective in eradicating the cancer. The role of additional chemo treatments is to extend the life of the patient, and what is wrong with that? A wonderful person and healthy in every other aspect can only want to live as long as life is enjoyable and useful. A seriously ill person will bargain for a few more years, months, then weeks, then a few days

The average milk production per cow in the top 24 states equaled 23,777 pounds of milk in 2020. That was an increase of 382 pounds per cow over 2019.

This equates to 2,764.8 gallons of milk per cow or an average of 9.2 gallons per day over the lactation period of 10 months or 300 days.

The density of milk is 8.6 pounds per gallon while the density of water is 8.3 pounds per gallon.

The number of high producing cows in the top 24 states was 9.5 million head in January of 2020. This was an increase of 16,000 milk cows from a year earlier, January 2019.

The average cow is milked about three years before being culled from the head.

The number of high producing cows is increasing and the milk production per cow is increasing. Milk production is still on the increase.

A high producing cow consumes 50-55 pounds of dry matter per day. The average dairy cow consumes about 40 gallons of quality water per day. The total water requirement for cleaning equipment and cleansing the animal, could be as high as 200 gallons per day per cow.

Summary of information on dairy cows in the top 24 states of the U.S.

Number of milk cows = 9.505 million (2021)

Pounds milk per cow per year = 23,777 (2020)

Gallons of milk per cow per day = 9.2

Gallons of milk per cow per year = 2,765

Density of milk is 8.6 pounds per gallon.

Density of water is 8.3 pounds per gallon.

Average cow is milked three years, then culled.

High producing cows may be milked 3 times daily or more.

Average cow consumes 40 gallons water/day.

Average water usage per cow, up to 200 gal./day.

Average size of dairy herd = over 300 milk cows.

Largest dairy herd = over 30,000 cows, Fair Oaks, IL. Rosedale Dairy Farms, 8,400 Wisconsin.

Current milk cow numbers are at an all-time high of 9.505 million cows, a 27 year high. Milk production has increased each year over the past 20 years.

Total milk production: 9.05 million x 23,777=225.9 billion pounds or 26.3 billion gallons. (an all-time record).

Production of milk in 2020 was 223 billion pounds, a 2 percent increase over 2019. Production of milk in 2000 was 167.4 billion pounds. Butter production is an all-time high.

The US Milk Farm Price received in 2022 was $24.30 per 100 pounds. The 2021 price was $17.60. This equates to 11.63 gallons of milk or $2 per gallon at the farm.

The top 10 states in number of milk cows (2021)

California	1.725 million cows
Wisconsin	1.263
Idaho	.635
New York	.626
Texas	.578
Pennsylvania	.483
Minnesota	.445
Michigan	.427
New Mexico	.330
Washington	.282

Chapter 11

CONNECTIONS BETWEEN MILK, DAIRY PRODUCTS AND CANCERS.

> Facts are stubborn things; and whatever may be our
> wishes, our inclinations, or the dictates of our passions,
> they cannot alter the state of facts and evidence.
>
> ....John Adams

The concentration of estrogen in milk is higher due to milking periods that extent long into the pregnancy, when concentrations of estrogens are highest. (8)

Estrogens from cow's milk have been studied in relation to the potential ill health effects, in particular, as regards the reproductive system. The incidence of breast cancer is rising in females (2) and likely ovarian cancer as well. (1,2).

Exogenous compounds (environmental pollutants) present in low concentrations could disrupt the development and function of the neuroendocrine system in vertebrates. Such compounds can affect hormonal receptors and thus disrupt cell signaling and homeostasis (8, 10) Sharpe and Skakkebeck (8) suggested an important source of estrogens was food of animal origin, especially milk and dairy products.

Exposure to exogenous estrogens as from milk is important to prenatal and prepubescent development of the reproductive system in children.

Endogenous levels of estrogens in children are low and any amounts of exogenous estrogens could interact with their hormonal system and disrupt the development of the urogenital tract, mammary glands and the central nervous system (8,11,13). Some of these disruptions could become evident only in adult life, even though they have an origin in prenatal or early postnatal disturbances in hormonal balance. Milk as a potential source of exogenous estrogens is especially important as consumption of cow's milk is usually the highest in children.

Exogenous estrogens could interfere with the normal function of estrogen receptors in the hypothalamus and pituitary gland, and also in peripheral, estrogen-responsive tissues (15).

Potential exposure to estrogens is especially important in regard to prenatal and prepubertal development of the reproductive system in children. Endogenous levels of estrogens in children could interact with their hormonal system and disrupt the development of the urogenital track, mammary glands and central nervous system evident in adult life.

The influence of exogenous estrogens on the endocrine system and cancer development has been reported in numerous studies and reviewed in many publications (11, 16 17). It should be noted that several pollutants, such as polychlorinated biphenyls (PCB's), or any other contaminants in the feed or grazing, with estrogenic properties, could be present in milk.

Risk of breast, prostate and development of the reproductive system (ovaries) exists from estrogen. The estrogen in dairy products is absorbed in the digestive tract where it is increased in blood levels and ultimately effects development of the reproductive system.

The milking period of a cow typically is extended into the eighth month of pregnancy. A cow typically will have about six weeks to 2 months prior to delivery of a calf when she is not milked. As production of estrogens by the placenta is increasing throughout the period of pregnancy, high levels of estrogen are in the milk. Estrogens are primarily synthesized in ovaries and the placenta. Estrogens as lipophilic substances easily pass through the blood-milk barrier and their presence in milk is in direct correlation with the levels in blood. (19)

Malekinejad et al. (25) have shown that during pregnancy cumulative concentrations of free and enzymatically deconjugated estrone (E1) increased from 7.9 ng/L in non-pregnant cows, to 1266 ng/L in the third trimester of pregnant cows. E2 increased from 18.6 to 51.2 ng/L over the same period. The concentration of conjugated estrogen estrone sulfate, increased up to 33 times during pregnancy.

Milk consumed today is different than milk consumed 100 years ago, especially in regards to concentration of different hormones, including estrogen and contaminants. Due mainly to improved selection and management of dairy herds, milk production per cow has increased about five-fold in the last 60 to 70 years (29).

Heat treatment (pasteurization) does not affect estrogens E1 and E2 concentrations. Souring does not affect concentration of estrogen in milk.

Production and consumption of milk and dairy products has vastly increased in the last decades due primarily to large commercial herds.

Estrogens in milk are present in free and in conjugated forms as sulfates and glucuroinates. Along with estrogens E1 and E2, the main estrogen in milk is estrone sulfate. Free, biologically active estrogens (E1 and E2) can be (re)formed from the estrone sulfate after consumption of cow's milk (16, 34). Orally ingested estrogens escape enterohepatic digestive processes and reach the systemic circulation directly, without passing through the liver (16, 35).

Low fiber diets may stimulate the absorption of estrogen from the digestive tract and increase the amount of exposure to estrogen.

The evidence that exposure to exogenous estrogens from various sources trigger cancer development in experimental animals is convincing. The carcinogenic effect of estrogens and some estrogens' metabolites is associated with an activation of estrogen receptors alpha and beta that stimulate transcription of genes promoting cell proliferation. (15) This physiological effect of estrogens during estrous cycle, pregnancy and lactation could also result in cancerous transformation of cells. Increased DNA replication could lead to increases in mutations occurring during DNA synthesis and estrogens could directly stimulate proliferation of different cells. Also, estrogens could stimulate the synthesis of various growth factors, which could stimulate proliferation of different cells through endocrine or paracrine mechanisms. (50) All these effects of estrogens could lead to cancer development, and the risk for cancer development increases with doses and length of exposure (15, 17) in both animals and humans.

Several female cancers such as breast cancer, ovarian cancer and uterine cancer are well known to be responsive to estrogens and in such cancers, one can easily imagine the connection between increased milk consumption and progression of the disease.

Higher availability of calcium in the body reduces the levels of vitamin D2. Vitamin D2 has been shown to have negative effects on cell proliferation and thus progressive development of neoplastic cells. (18)

In addition to sex steroid hormones, milk could contain several carcinogenic environmental pollutants such as dioxins, furans, pesticide residues, heavy metals and feed contaminants (phytoestrogens, mycotoxins (aflatoxin), which can also contribute to cancer development. There exists the potential synergistic effect of milk estrogens and environmental pollutants.

Incidence rates of breast, ovarian and uterine cancers with food intake in 40 countries showed high levels of milk intake were associated with the incidence of ovarian, endometrial, uterine and breast cancer.

Experiments in rats showed increased incidence of mammary tumors when fed low-fat milk. Consumption of estrone sulfate increased mammary tumor incidence.

Skimmed milk has the fat-soluble sex steroid hormones removed. Other manipulations of milk do not reduce the content of estrogens in milk.

https://eje.bioscientifica.com/view/journals/eje/179/6/EJE-18-0591.xml

References:

1. Manecksha RP and Fitzpatrick MJ. Epitemiology of testicular cancer. BJU International 2009 104 1329-1333. (https://doi.org/10. 1111/j.1464-410X 2009/08854.x)

2. Tao Z. et al. Breast cancer epidemiology and etiology. Cell Biochemistry and Biophysics 2015 72 333-336. (https://doi.org./10.1007/s12013-014-0459-6)

3. Sharpe, RM, Skakkebeak, NE. Are estrogens involved in falling sperm coiunts and disorders of the male reproductive tract? Lancet 1993 341 1392-1395. https://doi.org/10. 1016/0140-6736(93)90953-E)

4. Leon-Olea M et al. Current concepts in neuroendocrine disruption. General and Comparative endocrinology 2014 203 156-173. (https://doi.org/10.1016/j.ygcen/2014.02.005)

5. Andersson AM & Skakkebeck NE. Exposure to exogenous estrogens in food possible impact on human development and health. European Journal of Endocrinology 1999 140 477-485. (Https://doi.org/10.1530/eje.0.1400477)

6. Torfadottr JE et al. Milk intake in early life and risk of advanced prostate cancer. American Journal of Epidemiology 2012 175 144-153. (https://doi.org./10/1093/ake/kwr289)

7. Drobnis, EZ and Nangia AK. Male rerprloductive functions disrupted by pharmacological agents. Advances in Experimental Medicine and Biology 2017 1034 13-24. (https://doe.org/10.1007/978-3-319-69535-8_3)

8. Parodi PW. Impact of cow's milk estrogen on cancer risk. International Dairy Journal 2012 22 3-14. (Https://doi.org/10.1016/j.idairyj.2011.08.006)

9. Davoodi H, Esmaeili S & Martazavian AM. Effects of milk and milk products consumption on cancer: a review. Comprehensive Reviews in Food Science and Food Safety 2013 12 249-264. https://doi.org/10.1111/1541-4337.12011)

10. Pape-Zambito DA, Magliatro AL & Kensinger RS. 17B-Estradiol and estrone concentrations in plasma and milk during bovine pregnancy. Journal of Dairy Science 2008 91 127-135. https://doi.org/10.3169/jds.2007-0481)

11. Malekincjah H et al. Naturally occurring estrogens in processed milk and in raw milk (from gestated cows) Journal of Agriculture and Food Chemistry 2006 54 9785-97912. (https://doi.org/10 1021/jf061972e)

12. Capper JL et al. The environmental impact of dairy production: 1944 compared to 2007. Journal of Animal Science 2009 87 2160-2167. (https://doi.org/10/2527/ksd/2009-1781)

13. Macdonald IA, Bokkenheuser VD, Winter, J, McLemon AM, Misbach EH. Degradation of steroids in the human gut. Journal of Lipid Research. 1983 24 675700.-

14. Kuhnz W, Gansau C and Mahler M. Pharmascokinetics of estradiol, free and total estone, in young women following single intravenous and oral administration of 17 beta-estradiol. Arzneimitteelforschung 1993 43 966-973.

15. Key, TJA & Pike MC. The dose-effect relationship between unopposed estrogens and mitotic rate: its general role in explaining and predicting endometrial cancer risk. British Journal of Cancer 1988 57 205-212. (https://doi.org/10.1038bjc.1988.44)

16. Dickson RB & Lippman ME. Estrogenic regulation of growth and polypeptide growth factor secretions in human breast carcinoma. Endocrine Reviews 1987 8 29-43. (https://doi.org/10. 1210ediv-8-1-29)

17. Yue W, Santen RJ, Wang JP, Li Y, Verderame MF. Genotoxic metabolites of estradiol in breast: Potential mechanism of estradiol induced carcinogenesis. Journal of Steroid Biochemistry and Molecular Biology 2003 86 477-486. (Https://doi.org/10. 1016/ SO960-0760(03)00377-7)

18. Garland CF, et al. The role of vitamin D in cancer prevention. American Journal of Public Health 2006 96 252-261. (https://doi. org/10 2105Ajph 2004 045260)

19. Ganmaa D & Sato A. The possible role of female-sex hormones in milk from pregnant cows in the development of breast, ovarian and corpus uteri cancers. Medical Hypotheses 2005 65 1028-1037. (https:// doi.org/10.1016/j.mehy.2005.06.026)

Tomaz Snoj and Gregor Majdic. Mechanisms in Endocrinology: Estrogens in consumer milk: is there a risk to human reproductive Health? European Journal of Endocrinology. Vol 179. pp. R275-R286. 2018.

Chapter 11a

HORMONES, CONTAMINANTS IN MILK AND CANCER

The presence of hormones in milk and dairy foods was of concern in the past with respect to finding hormones as biomarkers in milk for disease and pregnancy diagnosis. Studies demonstrated that existing hormones in human and animal milk are essential for infant's growth and immunity.

More recently, evidence indicates that hormones as estrogen and insulin-like growth factors, are involved in tumors as endometrial breast, ovarian and prostate.

Cow's milk has the capability to mediate specific physiological and pathological functions. (1) The presence of hormones in dairy cow's milk has the capability to disrupt the physiological function of endocrine systems and this has raised concern worldwide. (2)

The most important hormones in milk and other dairy products consist of prolactin (PRL), steroids as estrogens, progesterone, corticoids, and androgens. Other hormones as insulin-like growth fctor-1 (IGF-1) (3) and local hormones including prostaglandins (PGs) (4,5) are in dairy products. PGs level in milk samples could be used as a marker of mastitis in cows. (5) The significance of this statement is a cause for pause.

Hormones in milk and dairy foods have biological effects on humans ranging from growth promoting effects to sex steroids, (6) to carcinogenic properties that associate to some active metabolites of oestrogens and IGF-1. (7)

Prolactin (PRL) is a polypeptide hormone found in milk of several species. (8) Subcutaneous injection of PRL in rat resulted in selective accumulation in milk glands. (9)

PRL is transported into the mammary epithelial cells by transcytosis and consequently released in the milk either in intact or cleaved forms. (10) The highest concentration of PRL found in milk of cows was during the first days following parturition (birth). (4) The best-established sites of PRL action in mammals is the mammary gland and ovaries. (11) Milk IGF-1 is not destroyed in milk by pasteurization, and is present in shelf milk. (3)

There is a significant positive correlation between cow's milk PGs concentration and somatic cell count. Healthy cows had 2.4 ng/ml while cows with mastitis had 3.4 ng/ml. (12) The presence of PGs in commercial milk of 3 ng/ml PGs was found in whole milk. (13) High levels of PGs in dairy milk could be considered as a marker for bacterial mastitis and other inflammations. (14)

Glucocorticoids (GCs) are hormones in cow's milk. The predominant glucocorticoid, cortisol, is taken up from the blood by the mammary glands of cows. (15,16)

Progesterones are largely produced in the ovaries and placenta. Progesterones are essential hormones in human and animal reproduction from ovulation to maintaining pregnancy, development of mammary glands and roles associated with sexual responsiveness. (17,18)

Progesterone is mainly distributed in cow's milk within the fat fraction of milk. (19) It is estimated that 60-80 percent of estrogens come from milk and dairy product in U.S. diets. (20)

Epidemiological studies indicate a strong relationship between cow's milk and dairy product consumption and incidence of testicular and prostate cancers. (21)

Progesterones in cow's milk and breast milk have been identified. (22) Pregnant dairy cows had the highest level of steroid hormones, especially oestrogen 18-Beta-oestradiol. (23)

Steroid hormones pass the blood-milk barrier to the mammary glands. The main estrogen in cow's milk is the biologically inactive 17 beta estradiol followed by 17 beta oestradiol. (24) The cumulative concentration of free and enzymatically deconjugated estrogens in the third trimester (1639 ng/L) was 27 times larger than in milk of cows in their first trimester of pregnancy (60ng/L). (25,26)

Japan has had a recent increase in milk consumption of about 20-fold and incidence of prostate cancer is increasing at the fastest rate in the world. (27)

Data have shown the high potency of estradiol as a growth factor in promoting cancers. Not only estradiol but its metabolites play a role in initiation of cancers. (28) Metabolites act as endogenous tumor initiators by formation of depurination (damage) to DNA adducts, the N-glycosidic bonds are cleaved to release the corresponding adenine or guanine from DNA. (29)

Receptor-mediated effects of estrogens including carcinogenesis conversion of estrogens also involves carcinogenesis. (29) Further metabolites bind to DNA and consequently form carcinogenic stable or depurinating DNA adducts. (30)

Estrogens have a carcinogenesis property and conversion of estrogens to catecholestrogens (CEs) involves carcinogenesis. (29).

Oestrogens are dose dependent. Girls have a higher concentration of oestrogens than boys which results in girls' maturation sooner than boys. (6)

Estrogen aids normal cell function and growth. Several different factors play a role in turning healthy cells to cancerous cells. When these factors exist, estrogen can at as a spark. The hormone causes cancer cells to multiply and spread.

There is an increasing body of evidence indicating properties of hormones in dairy products as possible impact on human health including the role of some estrogens and insulin-like growth factor in initiation and provoking breast, prostate and endometrial tumors.

The presence of steroid hormones in dairy products could be counted as an important risk factor for various cancers in humans. Prolactin (PRL) is a polypeptide hormone found in milk. (8) PRL is released from the anterior pituitary gland in response to milking stimuli. It is also found in many other glands.

Experimental studies demonstrated that subcutaneous injection of PRL in rat resulted in selective accumulation in milk glands. (9) Prolactin is transported into the mammary epithelial cells and consequently released in the milk either in tact or cleaved forms. (10) Highest concentration was in July and lowest in November, obviously somehow temperature related. (4)

The established sites of PRL in mammals include the mammary gland and ovaries. (11)

Treatment of lactating cows with bovine somatropin (bst) indicated a significant increase of milk IGF-1. The IGF-1 is a 70 amino acid-linked polypeptide was produced mainly by mammary glands.

Milk contains Glucocorticoids. Cortisol as the predominant glucocorticoid is taken from the blood by the mammary glands of cows. (15,16) Progesterone is largely produced in ovaries and placenta (17,18) and is distributed in the fat faction of milk. (19) As was shown earlier, 80 percent of estrogens come from milk and dairy products in western diets. (20) The oestrogen sulphate is the main conjugate in milk which has a relatively high oral bioactivity. (6) In addition to cancers as ovarian and breast, recent epidemiological studies indicate a very strong relationship between milk and dairy products with high consumption and high incidence of testicular and prostate cancers. (21)

Dairy cows are fed vegetal flours known to contain high amounts of phytoestrogens including isoflavones. There is a concern about the transfer of these compounds from the cow feed to the milk and finally to human food chain. (31) Phytoestrogens are capable to interact with both typical oestrogen receptors alpha and beta (32) and act as endocrine disruptors. Plant isoflavonoids as soybean products and other legumes are converted by intestinal bacteria to hormone-like compounds with estrogenic activity. (33) Existence of phytoestrogens in cow's milk has been identified. (22)

It is known that steroid hormones pass the blood-milk barrier and there is no doubt that they exist in milk. The presence of steroid hormones especially progesterone content in milk is used as a diagnostic tool of pregnancy. The distribution of estrogens, especially 17 beta oestradiol in fat or non-fat is controversial. Lopez et al. found no difference between whole milk and defatted milk. (34,35) A maximum concentration of total estrone (sum of free and conjugated forms) was found in butter of 1.47 nm/g, 11.3 times higher than in milk. (36)

All body tissues exert a response to estrogens. (37) Estrogen receptors and the involving enzymes in estrogen synthesis and metabolism have been identified in nearly all tissues. (38) The most sensitive section of human population to estrogens are children who are passing the prepubertal period and it is well known that despite the low concentrations of estrogens in this period, they play very crucial roles such as developing and growth during childhood. Early data has shown the high potency of estradiol as a growth factor in promoting cancers. Not only estradiol but its metabolites play a role in initiation of cancers. (28)

Cytochrome P450 monooxygenase oxidize the estradiol and oestrone into 2- or 4-catechol oestrogens. These two metabolites can also be methylated into methoxy-oestrogens by catechol-methyltransferase. Another metabolite pathway of oestrogens is formation of 16 alpha-hydroxyoestrone. Finally, the methoxyoestrogens may be converted into semiquinone and quinone, which previous studies demonstrated the latest metabolites can act as endogenous tumor initiators by formation of depurinating DNA adducts. (29)

There is an increasing body of evidence indicating the effect of dairy estrogens in tumor provoking or initiation and this evidence is of great concern. Increasingly veterinary drugs, especially growth promoting hormones utilized in veterinary medicine, result in an increase of the residues in milk and other dairy products.

Steroid hormones are potent compounds in dairy products and exert profound biological effects in humans. These compounds, even at low doses, have significant biological effects. It remains critical that the possible and potential impact of the present hormones, especially estrogens, in dairy products be clarified. Possible unwanted effects on human health by consumption of meat from oestrogen-treated animals cannot be excluded.

References:

1. Fitz-Gerald RJ, Murray BA, Walsh DJ. (2004). Hypotensive peptides from milk proteins. *J Nutr*, 134(4):980S-988S.
2. Servos MR, et al. (2005) Distribution of estrogens, 17beta-estradiol and estrone in Canadian municipal wastewater treatment plants. *Sci Total Environ*, 336)1-3):155-170.
3. Collier R, et al. (1991) Factors affecting insulin-like growth factor-1 concentration in bovine milk. *J Dairy Sci,* 74(9):2905-2911.
4. Schams, D, Karg H. (1987) Hormones in milk. *Ann N Y Acad Sci,* 464: 75-86.

5. Atroshi F, et al. (1987). Milk prostaglandins and 12. electrical conductivity in bovine mastitis. *Vet. Res Commun*, 11 (1): 15-22.

6. Andersson AM, Skakkeback NE. (1999) Exposure to exogenous estrogens in food: possible impact on human development and health. *Eur J Endocrinol*, 140(6):477-485.

7. Vadgama JV, et al. (1999). Plasma insulin-like growth factor-I and serum IGF-binding protein 3 can be associate with The progression of breast cancer, and predict the risk of recurrence and the probability of survival in African-American and Hispanic women. Oncology 57(4):330-340.

8. Yamamuro Y, Sensui N. (1980). Changes in prolactin bioactivity of milk following isolation from litter and oxytocin administration in rats. *Life Sci*, 60(11):809-815x.

9. Ryszka F, Doliska B, Suszka-Switek. (2002). Distribution of prolactin in selected rat organs and tissues. *Int J Tissue React*, 24(1):33-36.

10. Sinha YN. (1995) Structural variants of prolactin occurrence and physiological significance. *Endocr Rev*, 16(3):354-369.

11. Freeman ME, Kanyicska B, Leerant A, Nagy G. (2000) Prolactin: structure, function, and regulation of secretion. Physio Rev, 80(80):1523-1631.

12. Atroshi F, Parantainen J, Sankari S, Osterman T (1986) Postaglandins and glutathione peroxidase in bovine mastitis. *Res Vet Sci*, 40(3):361-366.

13. Materia AS, et al. (1984). Prostglandins in commercial *milk preparations. Their effect in the prevention of stress*-induced gastric ulcer. *Arch Surg*, 119(3):290-292.

14. Anderson IL, et al. (1985). Arachidonic acid metabolites in milk of cows during acute coliform mastitis. *Am J Vet Res*, 46(7):1573-1577.

15. Schwalm JW, Tucker HA. (1978). Glucocorticoids in mammary secretions and blood serum during reproduction and lactation and distributions of glucocorticoids, progesterone, and estrogens in fractions of milk. J Dairy Sci, 61(5):550-560.

16. Gorewit RC, Tucker A (1976) Comparison of binding proteins of glucocorticoids in mammary tissue and in blood sera from lactating cows. J Dairy Sci, 59(7):1247-1253.

17. Zalanyi S. (2001). Progesterone and ovulation. *Eur J Obstet Gynecol Reprod Biol*, 98(2)152-159.

18. Conneely OM et al. (2000) Reproductive functios of the progesterone receptor. J soc *Gynecol Investig*, 7:S25-32.

19. Gunzler O, et al. (1975). Practical experience in determing progesterone in milk for evaluation of fertility in the cow. *Tiearztl Umsch*, 30(3)111-118.

20. Renesar X, et al. (1999) Estrone in food: a factor influencing the development of obesity? *Eur J Nutr*, 38(5):247-253.

21. Gammaa D, et al. (2003). The experience of Japan as a clue to the etiology of testicular and prostatic caners. *Med Hypotheses*, 60(5):724-730.

22. Slavin JL. (1996). Phytoestrogens in breast milk-another advantage of breast-feeding? *Clin Chem*, 42(6 pt 1):841-842.

23. Hartmann S, Lacorn M, Steinhart H. Natural occurrence of steroid hormones in food. *Food Chemistry*, 62(1):7-20.

24. Erb RE, Chew BP, Keller HF. (1977) Relative concentrations of estrogen and progesterone in milk and blood, and excretion of estrogen in urine. *J Anim Sci*, 45(3):617-626.

25. 96-25. Wolford ST, Argoudelis CJ. (1979). Measurement of estrogens in cow's milk, human milk, and dairy products. J Dairy Sci, 62(9): 1458-1463.

26. Holdsworth RDJ, Heap RB, Booth JM, Hamon M. (1982). A rapid direct radioimmunossay for the measurement of oestone sulphate in the milk of dairy cows and its use in pregnancy diagnosis. J Endocrinol, 95(1):7-12.

27. Hsing AW, Tsao L, Devesa SS. (2000). International trends and patterns of prostate cancer incidence and mortality. *Int J Cancer*, 85(1):60-67.

28. Service RF. (1998) New role for estrogen in cancer? *Science*, 279(5357):1631-1633.

29. Cavalieri EL, et.al. (1997). Molecular origin of cancer:catechol estrogen-3,4-quinones as endogenous tumor initiators. *Proc Natl Acad Sci USA*, 94(20):10937-10942.

30. Bolton, JL, Shen L. (1996) p-Quinone methides are the major decomposition products of catechol estrogen o-quinones. *Carcinogenesis*, 17(5):925-929.

31. Antignac JP, et al. Identification of phytoestrogens in bovine milk using liquid chromatography/electrospray tandem mass spectrometry. *Rapid Commun Mass Spectrom*, 17(12):1256-1264.

32. Lelercq G, Jacquot Y. (2014). Interactions of isoflavones and other plant derived estrogens with estrogen receptors for prevention and treatment of breast cancer-considerations, concerning related efficacy and safety. JK Steroid *Biochem Mol Biol*, 139(1):237-44.

33. Adlercreutz CH. et al. (1995). Soybean phytoestrogen intake and cancer risk. *J Nutr*, 125 (3 suppl):757S-770S.

34. Abeyawardene SA, Hathorn DJ, Glencross RG. (1984). Concentrations of oestradiol-17 beta and progesterone in bovine plasma and defatted milk during the post-partum anovulatory period, during oestrous cycles and following ovarietomy. Br. Vet J, 140(5):458-467.

35. Lopez H, Bunch TD, Shipka MP. (2002) Estrogen concentrations in milk at estrus and ovulation in dairy cows. *Anim Reprod Sci*, 72 (1-2):37-46.

36. Hartmann S, Larkus M, Steinhart H. (1998). Natural occurrence of steroid hormones in food. *Food Chemistry*, 62 (1): 7-20

37. Daxenberger A, Ibarreta D, Meyer HH. (2001). Possible health impact of animal oestrogens in food. *Hum Reprod Update*. 7 (3): 340-355.

38. Sharpe RM, Turner KJ, Sumpter JP. (1998) Endocrine disruptors and testis development. *Environ Health Perspect*, 106 (5): A220-221.

Chapter 12

MILK, DAIRY PRODUCTS, AND HEALTH.

The bottom line about milk and dairy products in general, is **that they are not necessary in the diet for optimal health**. Milk consumption is primarily limited to Caucasians because of lactose intolerance.

Lactose intolerance is common in the U.S., as it affects 95 percent of Asian Americans, 74 percent of Native Americans, 70 percent of African Americans, 53 percent of Mexican Americans, and 15 percent of Caucasians. When people so affected consume milk, typical symptoms are upset stomach, diarrhea, and gas, perhaps long-term medical problems as well.

Many people in the U.S. have a high incidence of lactose intolerance and do not want to take the risk of illness from dairy products. There are many sources of food that supply the nutrients found in milk. Milk is about 88 percent water of which consumers pay a high price. Compare the diet of Caucasians in the U.S. to the diet of people in the rest of the world, and indeed, all other mammalians, and it will be found that Caucasians are about the only adult group who consume milk to any great extent.

Infants and all mammalians require milk when first born and until they are capable of eating foods that supply needed nutrients. They produce enzymes (lactase) that digest the sugar (lactose) in the milk of the mother. When a child or a young animal becomes of age to eat adult food, they no longer have a requirement to nurse. After weening, often forced upon the young by the mother, needed nutrition is supplied by a non-dairy diet and the subject becomes naturally lactose intolerant, meaning they no longer digest the milk sugar lactose in milk.

Research has shown that dairy products have little or no benefit for bone health. A British medical journal article stated that most studies fail to show any link between dairy intake and bone fractures, including stress fractures. The study involved 96,000 young males and concluded that the more milk they consumed as teenagers, the more bone fractures they experienced as adults. This has largely been determined to be due to the casein proteins in milk.

Lactose activity decreases precipitously after about age five in children, leading to lactose intolerance in most populations. This occurs because the mammalian body is designed to wean the offspring off of mother's milk and be sustained by adult food. The majority of those who are not lactose intolerant are called lactase persistent (lactase, the enzyme that digests the sugar in milk).

Lactose intolerance is the prevalent genetic deficiency syndrome worldwide and it affects more than about 70 percent of the world population.

People who are lactose intolerant do not digest the milk sugar lactose and lactase deficiency leads to improper digestion of lactose. The undigested lactose travels from the small intestine into the colon (large intestine), dragging massive amounts of water through a process called osmosis, which can lead to watery diarrhea. The undigested lactose gets metabolized by bacteria in the colon, resulting in fermentation, which produces copious amounts of gases as hydrogen, carbon dioxide, and the foul-smelling sulfur gas.

There are a number of symptoms of lactose intolerance following consumption of milk: abdominal distention (bloating), cramps, abdominal pain, excessive flatulence (gas), diarrhea, burping, acid reflux and constipation. These symptoms may occur 30 minutes to two hours following consumption of dairy products. Lactose intolerance may be misdiagnosed as Irritable-Bowel- Syndrome (IBS).

Lactose intolerance may also be interpreted for dairy sensitivity which is an allergic reaction to the proteins (casein) in dairy products that lead to eczema, sinus problems, allergic reactions of the gastrointestinal lining, worsening of inflammatory bowel disease, and other allergic conditions. One may become lactose intolerant with aging.

Milk intolerance could also occur after intestinal infections or inflammatory conditions such as rotavirus, infection, Crohn's disease, celiac disease, radiation therapy, a giardia (an intestinal infection caused by a giardia parasite), and other medical issues.

The best way to diagnose lactose intolerance is to avoid all dairy products for at least 30 days. Labels must be reviewed as dairy products are in many packaged foods. If the symptoms recur following the reintroduction of dairy products in the diet, the best solution is to eliminate dairy from the diet.

There are four major dietary carbohydrates: lactose, fructose, sucrose, and starch. The enzyme lactase is found in the lining of the small intestine wall. When the lactose sugar is digested it forms two molecules of simple sugars, glucose and galactose. These sugars are absorbed through the intestinal wall into the blood vessels. Glucose is the sugar thought to feed all 37.2 billion human cells. Galactose is a highly suspicious sugar and it is disturbing what effect the sugar galactose might have on ovarian cancer.

The lactose persistent population is typically Northern "European" descent. This culture domesticated the cow and milked cows up to 4,000 years ago. There was a period of about 4,500 years when Europeans could not consume dairy products because of lactose intolerance. About 4,000 years ago, about 230 nomadic herders from Russia's Great Steppes migrated to northern Europe. The people were called Anatolian farmers who had begun to raise cattle 6,500 B.C. They soon had offspring who carried the genes to produce the enzyme lactase. Their offspring became milk drinkers as adults. In the frigid winters, the cow supplied fat, protein and meat. This was a time when other foods likely were not available. What the cow was fed and what she consumed for quality water will always be questionable. The cow has the ability to consume the dead forages of winter and convert them to milk and meat. Snow was available for consumption for water.

The dairy lobby is one of the most influential in Washington, D.C. The dairy lobbies assist dairies with large commercial herds exploiting tax breaks and benefits to dominate the market place. Small farms are dying.

The US dairy industry is the taxpayer bankrolling the delusions of prominent agribusiness. Dairy is a dying industry. "Let Dairy Die" is a campaign driven by Direct Action Everywhere (DxE), an alliance of animal rights activists.

In 2018, seven percent of dairies shut down. None of the government subsides focus on getting farmers out of dairy production.

Additional thoughts: Don't drink milk for health. Countries with the highest intake of dairy products invariably are the countries with the most osteoporosis. Cow's milk is a deterrent to good bone health because of caseins in the protein of the milk. It is thought the caseins in the milk actually are the cause of osteoporosis and poor bone strength.

Whole Milk is made up of fat (3.5-4.0%) and protein suspended in water. Light scatters and reflects a white color.

In a January, 2008 article titled "The Milk Letter: A Message to My Patients published on the AFPA Fitness Website, Robert M. Kradjian, MD, Surgeon at Seton Medical Centre, wrote:

"You may be horrified to learn that the USDA allows milk to contain from one to one and a half million white blood cells per milliliter (That's 1/30 of an ounce). If you don't already know this, I'm sorry to tell you that another way to describe white blood cells where they don't belong would be to call them pus cells." (The white blood cell count has since been reduced to 750,000 cells per milliliter.)

Monsanto Sued by University of California over patent rights for BST

Three researchers at the University of California, San Francisco, were the first to isolate and identify the genetic code for bovine growth hormone (BGH). The University sued Monsanto in February 2004, after it had received one of its patents. The patent claims a DNA comprising deoxynucleotide sequence coding for bovine growth hormone. The patent was originally filed in August 1980 and again filed February 15, 1990. The University of California received patent number 6,692,941 in February 2004. Monsanto was able to reach an agreement with the University of California as the case was set to begin a jury trial.

The FDA approved Monsanto's recombinant bovine growth hormone (rBGH) product, Posilac, for commercial use on November 5, 1993. The rBGH Posilac is a genetically engineered bovine somatotropin (BST). Posilac was sold following a 90-day moratorium on the sale of rBGH on February 3, 1994. Posilac was sold 10 years before the UC patent was issued.

The University of California patent claims had been pending for 24 years. Monsanto agreed to pay the University of California $100 million dollars, and an ongoing royalty of 15 cents per dose of Posilac sold, with a minimum royalty of $5 million annually until 2023, or at least an additional $95 million. It was estimated that about one-third of dairy cows were receiving Posilac shots every two weeks in 2008. The shots sell for 25-70 cents each.

As part of the settlement, Monsanto was granted an exclusive license to the University's patents for making recombinant bovine growth hormone (rBGH).

Posilac injected into cows is intended to have cows produce more milk, an estimated 10-20 percent more. This then is the intent of cows to produce more milk from a given amount of feed. It is known that one of the issues with using Posilac is increased infection of the mammary glands, resulting in increased mastitis (pus). This likely is at least partially responsible for the short life-span of high producing dairy cows.

As of April 13, 2022 Bovine somatotropin (BST), also known as bovine growth hormone (BGH), is an animal drug approved by FDA to increase milk production in dairy cows. The rBST is carried to the liver where it stimulates the liver to produce insulin-like Growth Factor (IGF-1), a protein hormone that aids in turning nutrients into milk. The IGF-1 is transferred to the cow's mammary gland where it stimulates milk production.

The FDA approved the label insert for Posilac (the Monsanto brand Artificial Bovine Growth Hormone 'BGH'). Monsanto admits that its 'use is associated with increased frequency of use of medication in cows for mastitis and other health problems.' Monsanto's own data further show that up to an 80% incidence of mastitis, an udder infection, in hormone-treated cattle resulting in contamination of milk with statistically significant levels of pus.

Samuel S. Epstein was a prolific writer and authored the book, "What's in your Milk?" Dr. Epstein conducted a 20-year fight against "cancer causing milk."

Samuel S. Epstein, MD, Chairman of the Cancer Prevention Coalition, wrote in a March 20, 1994 article "A Needless Risk of Breast Cancer," published in the Los Angeles Times. Dr. Epstein pointed out the potential cancer from milk. (Dr. Epstein has also written on the politics of cancer.)

We will see how the "gang" responded to negative information to the dairy industry by attacking Dr. Epstein.

"It was a egregious disservice to all consumers, and especially women concerned about breast cancer, for the times to have provided a forum for Samuel S. Epstein's widely rejected attacks on the safety of bovine somatotropin (BST). (anonymous)

The American Cancer Society issued a statement declaring: Extensive testing and research has shown that rBST is indistinguishable from natural bovine growth hormone and thus entails **no** risk for consumers. There are no valid scientific findings to indicate a risk of human carcinogenesis. (Note the use of the word "no" in their message. (…please sent a huge donation!)

The Food and Drug Administration was equally direct.

"Claims that IGT-1 in milk could result in premature development of breasts in young children and breast cancer in adults are not only not substantiated in the scientific literature, but in fact have no basis in science." (Consider where the money comes from to sponsor research on milk, cancer, and so many subjects that are subject to the politics of the system.)

Virginia V. Weldon, M.D., Monsanto's Senior Vice President (Monsanto produces BST, and milk is an important commerce product for Monsanto) wrote: "In short, neither BST nor IGF-1 poses any breast cancer health risk. But in printing Epstein's latest pseudoscientific charge The Times has caused untold scores of women to mistakenly believe something is dangerously wrong with their milk. The 'needless new risk' as your paper titled the article, isn't BST or IGF-1-it's the misinformation promoted by newspapers that are either unwilling or unable to determine the veracity of the facts they provide their readers." (Note the use of the word "any". This was to send a message to newspapers not to print articles that contain scientific information deleterious to the wishes of the "machine".)

Researchers who go against the "flow" will also be ostracized. It would appear all of the above would have to sign off on research before it could be published relating to dairy products as well as many forms of cancer.

This likely is why there has been so little research on milk and milk products in the past quarter century, especially as relates to dairy products and their effect on the initiation of cancer.

There are any number of articles available describing the treatment of cows and discussion of the quality of milk at the farm level. Milk is blended from farm to farm before being processed. Some articles might leave you with such deterrence that one would like to never drink milk or eat dairy products again. If the potential for impurities and disease means anything, one might decide that milk and dairy products are something not needed in a wholesome diet.

The largest dairy company in the U.S. is Dairy Farmers of America, Inc. In 2019, this firm had sales of $11.361 billion of dairy products and a market share of 11.9 percent.

In 2019, the U.S. produced over 218 billion pounds of milk, 25.35 billion gallons. Milk consumption in the U.S. has decreased from about 198 pounds/capita in 2000 to 141 pounds/capita in 2020, about a 29 percent decrease.

The 15 largest U.S. dairies:

1.	Dairy Farms of America, Inc.	$11.4 billion
2.	Nestle USA	$11.0 billion
3.	Danone North America	$ 6.5 billion
4.	Schreiber Foods, Inc.	$ 5.0 billion
5.	Kraft Heinz Co.	$ 4.9 billion
6.	Conagra Brands	$ 4.6 billion
7.	Prairie Farms Dairy	$ 4.2 billion
8.	Land O'Lakes	$ 4.0 billion
9.	California Dairies	$ 4.0 billion
10.	Unilever, N. Amer. Op.	$ 3.9 billion
11.	Glanbia Nutrition	$ 3.5 billion
12.	Leprino Foods Co.	$ 3.5 billion
13.	The Kroger Co.	$ 3.3 billion
14.	Great Lakes Cheese	$ 3.2 billion
15.	Lactalis Group N.A. Op.	$ 3.0 billion

(Medical doctors have been vocal about the detrimental effects wrought by milk consumption and inclusion of dairy products in daily diets!)

Chapter 13

ANTIOXIDANTS AND CANCER

Antioxidants are compounds that inhibit oxidation. Oxidation is a chemical reaction that can produce free radicals and chain reactions that damage the cells. Antioxidants are often described as "mopping up" of free radicals. Antioxidants can be used to inhibit oxidation to counteract the deterioration of stored food products as well.

Free radicals are highly reactive and unstable molecules that are naturally produced within the body via metabolism when converting food to energy. Environmental sources as pollutants in the air and water and sunlight may be an additional source of production of free radicals.

Free radicals may cause oxidative stress, a process that can trigger cell damage. Oxidative stress is thought to play a role in a variety of diseases as cancer, cardiovascular diseases, diabetes, Alzheimer's disease, Parkinson's disease, and eye diseases such as cataracts and age-related macular degeneration.

Free radicals are produced naturally in the body, and they do have a purpose. All free radicals are not bad. They can help fight infection, help repair tissue injury, and attack invaders in the blood. They also assist the immune system.

A poor diet, too much exercise, and high emotional or physical stress can produce harmful free radicals.

Free radical damage can cause deterioration of the collagen, elastin fibers and DNA within the cells and they can accelerate cell death. Aging slows down and stops the production of collagen and elastin causing the weak and damaged skin to lose elasticity, plumpness, and moisture causing fine lines, wrinkles, saggy skin, texture irregularities, and dryness. Dead cells stay on the surface of the skin longer as the cell turnover rate slows. The question, what can one do to reverse this action?

Antioxidants in the diet can neutralize unstable free radicals by donating an electron and ending the electron-stealing chain reaction that causes oxidative stress.

One of the ways to minimize free radical damage is to eat a diet rich in antioxidants. The list of foods is long; berries, cherries, citrus (especially oranges), prunes, garlic and onions, cinnamon, foods rich in vitamins A, C, and E. Whole grains, nuts, seeds, and wheat germ provide antioxidants. This is not a complete list. Living a healthy life style goes along with eating right. Minimize high fructose in the diet, and other sugars, excess fat, artificial flavorings, preservatives and synthetic or processed food.

High dose supplements of antioxidants may be linked to health risks, interacting with body enzymes and medications. Food is a safe source of antioxidants. Vegetables and fruits are healthy foods and rich sources of antioxidants. There is no evidence that antioxidant supplements can prevent cancer or other diseases.

Free radicals are highly reactive unstable molecules that are produced in the body naturally as a byproduct of normal metabolism, or by exposure to toxins in the environment as ultraviolet light. Free radicals have a lifespan of only a fraction of a second, but during that time they can damage DNA, sometimes resulting in mutations that can lead to various diseases, including heart disease and cancer.

Free radicals are atoms that contain an unpaired electron. Due to this lack of a stable number of outer shell electrons they are in a constant search to bind with another molecule to stabilize themselves, a process that can cause damage to cells. This damage may accelerate the aging process and can play a role in the development of cancer and other diseases.

There are many types of free radicals. In humans, the most significant are oxygen free radicals (reactive oxygen species). Examples include single oxygen (when oxygen is "split" into single atoms with unpaired electrons), hydrogen peroxide, superoxide, and hydroxyl anions.

The production of free radicals in normal metabolic processes along with radon, asbestos, vinyl chloride, some viruses, air pollution; are among the factors that the risk of many different diseases increase with age, even when people have few direct exposures to disease-causing substances.

Radon is emitted from the normal decay of uranium in the soil that gets trapped in homes. Radon is the second leading cause of lung cancer behind smoking.

Once free radicles are generated through exposure to a carcinogen (a substance capable of causing cancer in living tissue) or during the normal processes of body metabolism, they are free to do damage.

Carcinogens initiate cancer by damaging DNA that carries genetic information to the cells. The damaged DNA may result in mutations. These lead to a disruption in the normal process of growth and cell division. Cells divide more quickly with an increase in the possibility of a cancerous cell developing.

The ability of a carcinogen to cause cancer depends upon several factors. The most obvious are the amount and length of time of exposure. Individual health and other personal factors as age that either raise or lower risk of cancer.

Cancer is most often caused by an accumulation of situations, rather than a single situation. A number of factors may work together to either increase or decrease the risk of developing cancer. When there is damage to the DNA, the body produces proteins that repair damaged DNA or eliminate damaged cells before a normal cell is transformed into a cancer cell. There are tumor suppressor genes that slow down cell division and conduct repairs.

Free radicals are highly unstable atoms that can damage cellular DNA, which is thought to play a role in the development of cancer. Free radicals roam around the body and can cause inflammation. Antioxidants work by tracking down free radicals, and neutralizing their harmful effects.

The availability of free radicals creates what is known as oxidative stress on the body. The reason for the term oxidative stress is that the chemical reactions that result in free radicals obtaining an electron are done in the presence of oxygen.

The process can involve a series of reactions. When one free radical "steals" an electron from a molecule, that molecule becomes a free radical because it is missing an electron and so on. Free radicals can damage the body's DNA, which contains genes, as well as proteins, lipids, cell membranes and more.

Damage done to genes in the DNA may result in genes that produce ineffective proteins; some of these proteins are watch keepers over the DNA integrity.

Tumor suppressor genes code for proteins that function to repair damages in DNA or cause cells that are damaged beyond salvage to be removed through a process of apoptosis (programmed cell death). Most often, it is a series of mutations in tumor suppressor genes and other genes that leads to the formation of a cancer cell.

Many of the phytochemicals (plant chemicals) in the foods we eat function as antioxidants. These nutrients function by inhibiting the formation of free radicals that may reduce the damage they would cause in the body. This is thought to be at least part of the reason why a diet rich in vegetables and fruits have been linked with a lower risk of human diseases.

Cancer cells are different from normal cells in how they grow and look. The normal cell has to go through many steps to become a cancerous cell.

The major differences between normal cells and cancer cells relate to growth, communication, cell repair and size. Normal cells have "stickiness", do not spread from their assigned location. This is an important concept that holds normal cells in place. Cancer cells to not have this stickiness and can float freely to new areas in the body. A special difference between the two types of cells.

Whereas normal cells stop when there are enough cells, cancer cells continue to grow uncontrolled. Normal cells respond to signals from other cells, whereas, cancer cells do not. Cancer cells do not replace aged or damaged cells. Normal cells are repaired or replaced and stay together in assigned areas. Cancer cells are not replaced or repaired and can travel solo throughout the body.

Normal cells look uniform under a microscope whereas cancer cells are varied in size, larger and darker centered. Normal cells reach maturity, before designated tasks, blood vessels grow to feed normal growth and aid in repair. Cancer cells do not reach maturity and divide before reaching maturity, can "hide" and can grow uninterrupted. Cancer cells control blood vessel growth to feed tumors.

Each gene in the body carries a blueprint that codes for a different protein. Some of these proteins are growth factors, chemicals that tell cells to grow and divide, etc.

If the gene that codes for one of these proteins is stuck in the "on" position by a mutation (an oncogene). the growth factor proteins continue to be produced.

Homeostasis is the body's way of ensuring all its processes are working properly. Homeostasis normal cells either repair or die (undergo apoptosis) when they are damaged or get old. Cancer cells are not repaired nor do they die.

The gene p53 has the job of checking to see if a cell is too damaged to repair, and if so, advise the cell to kill itself. If this p53 protein is abnormal or inactive from a mutation in the p53 gene, then old or damaged cells are allowed to reproduce and undergo apoptosis.

The p53 gene is one type of tumor suppressor gene that code for proteins that suppress the growth of cells.

Normal cells secrete substances that make them stick together in a group. Cancer cells do not make these substances and can "float away" to locations nearby, or through the bloodstream or system of lymph channels to distant regions in the body, metastasize.

When cancer cells arrive in a new region (such as lymph nodes, the lungs, the liver, or the bones), they begin to grow, often forming tumors far removed from the original tumor.

It was noted that cancer cells exhibit much more variability than normal cells in cell size, larger and smaller, and an abnormal shape, both the cell and nucleus (the brain of the cell). The nucleus appears both larger and darker than normal cells. The reason for the darkness is the nucleus of cancer cells contain excess DNA. Cancer cells often have an abnormal number of chromosomes arranged in a disorganized fashion.

Proto-oncogenes are a group of genes that cause normal cells to become cancerous when they are mutated. The mutated version of a proto-oncogene is an oncogene. Even when DNA cells are damaged and mutations occur to convert a proto-oncogene to an oncogene, many of these cells are repaired. The tumor suppressor genes are proteins that function to repair damaged DNA or eliminate damaged cells.

These proteins help reduce the risk of cancer even when an oncogene is present. If mutations in the suppressor genes are also present, the likelihood of cancer developing is greater as abnormal cells are not repaired and continue to survive instead of undergoing apoptosis (programmed cell death). Many changes are needed to transform a normal cell to a cancer cell. Changes in the cell that prolong survival of deranged cells, changes that grow and divide uncontrollably, and fail to respond to normal signals for cells to die, fail to respect boundaries with other cells (lose contact inhibition) and other characteristics that cause cancer cells to behave different than normal cells.

Most oncogenes regulate the proliferation of cells, but some inhibit differentiation (process of cells becoming unique types of cells) or promote survival of cells (inhibit programmed death). Proteins produced by some oncogenes work to suppress the immune system, reducing the chance that abnormal cells will be recognized and eliminated by immune cells such as T-cells. Cancer cells tend to have mutations that can affect a number of processes in the growth of the cell.

The cells of the bone marrow, undergo cell division more rapidly than those of any organ in the system and are particularly vulnerable to damage from a cytotoxic dose.

Chemotherapeutic agents act principally on dividing cells. Bone marrow depression is a side-effect of nearly all such drugs and is the dose-limiting side effect of most.

Cardiac damage is the dose-limiting toxicity of anthracycline group of antitumor antibiotics related to anthraquinones and can cause cumulative cardiomyopathy. Damage to the liver is a complication of many drugs.

Kidney toxicity is being increasingly recognized and may be dose-limiting. Kidneys are vulnerable to damage from chemotherapeutic agents as they are the elimination pathway for many drugs and their metabolites. One of the first indications of damage to kidneys is discovery of proteins in the urine. Severe problems follow-on when the kidneys cannot remove excess potassium known as hyperkalemia. Hyperkalemia can be a recurrent condition and poses an increased risk of mortality. (Could have well been what killed Celeste). When there is a breakdown or destruction of cells, the electrolyte potassium moves from inside the cell to outside the cell wall. This shift of potassium outside of the cells causes hyperkalemia. Extreme stress is placed upon the heart under these circumstances.

Tumor lysis syndrome, occurs when receiving chemotherapy or other drug treatments. the drugs will act by breaking down the tumor cells. Then there could be a rapid amount of cellular destruction, the components of the cells (including potassium), will move outside of the cell, and into the blood stream. A blood test will reflect high potassium. A normal potassium level is 3.5-5.0 millimoles per liter or mmol/L. Having a blood potassium level higher that 6.0 mmol/L can be life-threatening and may require immediate treatment. A reading as high as 7 mmol/L has been noted when being treated for cancer and this reading may reoccur even after receiving the best medical attention along with hospitalization. A spike of potassium of a reading of 7.0 mmol/L requires immediate medical assistance at the emergency of the hospital. (The potassium spiked to 7.0 mmol/L three times for Celeste when hospitalization was required).

Chapter 13a

ASPIRIN

Aspirin is known as a salicylate and a nonsteroidal anti-inflammatory drug (NSAID). This medication is effective by stopping blood platelets from clumping together and forming blood clots, the cause of heart attack and stroke. Aspirin is long-lasting and may not be effective immediately. A crystal form of aspirin dissolves rapidly and would be a better choice in the event of a heart attack, stroke or instant pain relief. Aspirin is an acid and should be taken with a full glass of water. It is suggested that one should not lie down for at least 10 minutes after taking aspirin. One should not lie down after suffering a heart attack but sit up. Aspirin is also taken for fever and/or inflammation. It should not be taken with another NSAID. It should not be taken with alcohol. A doctor should be notified if any unusual symptoms occur.

Production of a drug called *"aspirin"* began in 1897. The acetylsalicylic acid is a novel organic compound that does not occur in nature. It was first successfully synthesized in 1897. Scientists at the drug and dye firm Bayer began investigating acetylated organic compounds as possible new medicines, following the success of acetanilide ten years earlier. The name *Aspirin* was Bayer's brand name, rather than a generic name of a drug. Bayer could not patent the drug in Germany as it was declared ineligible. It was patented in the U.S. Patent number 644,077 issued 27 February 1900. In 1903, Bayer set up an American solidary. A patent was filed in Britain 22 December 1998 but was overturned in 1905.

Edward Stone, an English chaplain, had tasted the bark of willow tree in 1758 and noticed an astringency reminiscent of Peruvian bark, which was used to treat malaria. In 1763, Stone sent a letter to the Royal Society and described the dramatic power of powdered white willow bark to cure intermittent fevers.

In 1828 Johann Buchner obtained relatively pure salicin crystals from willow bark. A year later, Henri Leroux developed a procedure for extracting modest yields of salicin. In 1834, Swiss pharmacist Johann Pagenstecher discovered a new pain-reducing substance, isolated from meadowsweet, Filipendula ulmaria. By 1838, Italian chemist Raffaele Piria discovered a method of obtaining a more potent acid from of willow extract, which he named salicylic acid. The German chemist Karl Jacob Lowig had been working to identify the *Spiraea* extract. He soon realized that it was the same salicylic acid that Piria had found.

In 1876, the Scottish physician Thomas MacLagan experimented with salicin as a treatment for acute rheumatism, with considerable success. He reported the study in the Lancet. By the 1880s, the German chemical industry developed dyes from coal tar and was investigating new tar-derived medicines. In 1894, chemist Felix Hoffman joined the Bayer team. Hoffman's chemical success, diacetylmorphine, branded as heroin because of the heroic feeling it gave them. Felix Hoffman is named on the U.S. Patent as the inventor of aspirin, although a number of others in the Bayer company made large contributions to the development and success of aspirin

The name Aspirin was derived from the name of the chemical in German, Acetylspirsaure. Spirsaure (salicylic acid) was named for the meadowsweet plant, *Spirea ulmaria*, from which it could be derived. The -a is for acetylation, -spir- from Spirsaure, and added –in as a typical drug name ending to make it easy to pronounce.

After the U.S. declared war on 'Germany in April 1917, the U.S. seized all of Bayer's American holdings. After the Trading with the Enemy Act was amended, it allowed sale of the Rensselaer, New York plant and all of Bayer's American patents and trademarks, including the Bayer cross logo. In 1994, the rights to Bayer Aspirin and the U.S. rights to the Bayer name and trademarks were sold back to Bayer AG for US $1billion. Sterling Products, Inc. had owned all of the Bayer name and trademarks.

Alka-Seltzer is a soluble mix of aspirin and bicarbonate of soda.

In 1946, scientists at Yale found a substance to be the metabolically active derivative of acetanilide: acetaminophen. It was marketed by Bayer as Panadol in 1956. *Tylenol* pills were available in 1956 and by 1967 were available without a prescription. In 1962, ibuprofen was sold as Motrin in the U.S. In the 1980s ibuprofen became available without a prescription. Aspirin had a lot of competition.

In the early 1980s Reye's syndrome, a potentially fatal disease, surfaced by a suggested link between children's consumption of Bayer Aspirin.

In 1958 it was verified that aspirin works locally to combat pain and inflammation. In a 23 June paper in the journal *Nature,* it was suggested that aspirin and similar drugs (the nonsteroidal anti-inflammatory drugs or NSAIDs) worked by blocking the production of prostaglandins (note cancer connection). Later research showed that NSAIDs such as aspirin worked by inhibiting cyclooxygenase, (note cancer connection), the enzyme responsible for converting arachidonic acid into prostaglandin.

In the 1960s aspirin was known to have an anti-adhesive effect on blood platelets and aspirin had a low toxicity effect. By 1963 the anti-thrombosis effect of aspirin was known.

In 2019, the American Heart Association and American College of Cardiology changed clinical practiced guidelines, recommending against the routine use of aspirin in people older than 70 years of age or people with increased bleeding risk who do not have existing cardiovascular disease. (I do not personally believe the reasons are based on good evidence and will continue to take an aspirin daily!)

About 50 years ago, I was having vision problems. A dark veil would close over my eyes periodically without warning. When driving an auto I would have to pull off of the road and wait for a period when the problem vanished.

I visited a medical clinic in Minneapolis, MN where five trained physicians from the famed eye clinic in Miami, FL were located.

Following a diagnostic examination, the physician reminded me that as a young man I had migraine headaches, which I had forgotten. His recommendation was for me to take a 325 mg aspirin daily. When I forget to take the aspirin, "stars" appear in my vision path. Taking an aspirin clears up my problem. This has been going on for nearly 50 years. Am I a deserved advocate of aspirin for a good reason?

Aspirin is a safe and inexpensive drug that can effectively inhibit the enzyme COX-2. The C0X-2 enzyme converts unsaturated fatty acids into prostaglandins. Aspirin directly inhibits the release of free fatty acids into the bloodstream (lipolysis). Aspirin inhibits the enzyme responsible for the synthesis of cortisol. Aspirin prevents production of prostaglandins, inhibits cortisol production and lipolysis, it negates the direct estrogenic, anti-thyroid and immunosuppressive effects of unsaturated fatty acids.

It seems aspirin has much to offer as a low-cost drug to enhance health. In general, there will not be great support from the medical side of the street for aspirin. Let your doctor explain why! (If he /she can).

Source: https://en.m.wikipedia.org/wiki/History_of_aspirin

Chapter 14

JOE TIPPENS STORY

Joe Tippens is a financial strategist and executive with over 30 years working in the financial arena. He was CEO of Strategic Capital Group LLC and SCG Advisors LLV (Vero Beach, FL) an investment management firm he co-founded.

He was from a small town in Oklahoma and attended Oklahoma State.

Joe Tippens was diagnosed with stage IV small cell lung cancer in September 2016. He immediately went to MD Anderson Cancer Clinic in Houston, TX.

Chemo and radiation were started simultaneously. He had a large tumor in his left lung. Following treatment, he had less than one percent survivability and a median/mean life expectancy of three months. His initial weight went from 200 to 115.

Joe returned to Oklahoma and contacted a veterinarian. He was informed that a scientist in Merck Animal Health had performed cancer research on mice by injecting them with different types of cancers into different body parts. A product was discovered in their canine product line that was effective in killing these cancers.

The Merck researcher was diagnosed with stage IV brain cancer and was given a short time to live. She decided to take the same canine medication that was effective with the mice cancers. Six weeks later, she was cancer free.

The product is Safe-Guard Canine Dewormer.

Joe took the Canine Dewormer and also took Curcumin, GBD, and Vitamin E starting in January 2017. He has since dropped Vitamin E.

He took the above treatments daily and the Dewormer three consecutive days per week. He was receiving 222 milligrams of fenbendazole, the active ingredient in Dewormer.

In July 2020 he changed the fenbendazole to seven days a week, 222 milligrams per dose with a meal.

He suggests take this medication while on chemo or radiation treatments.

Joe Tippens is free of cancer as verified by CT scan. He says he will be on fenbendazole the rest of his life as he fears the cancer could come back.

That is the story of Joe Tippens.

I read this story and we decided that Celeste should try this treatment.

We started the fenbendazole and alternative treatments on October 24, 2021. By November 10 when we were notified that there would be no more chemo treatments, Celeste had taken 18 doses.

When the cancer treatments were discontinued, we doubled the dose rate to twice daily. By November 30 she had taken 51 doses.

We were very optimistic and conversed about how wonderful it would be if no one had to worry about cancer again. We were sure the next CA-125 blood test would be in the "normal" range.

A blood test revealed that the CA-125 reading had further increased to over 800. By this time Celeste had taken 74 doses of the fenbendazole and the alternative treatments. At three doses a week, this would be the equivalent of 25 weeks of treatment. It was obvious neither the fenbendazole nor the alternative treatments were working.

What worked for Joe Tippens did not work for Celeste. It is not that I doubt anything about Joe Tippens. Not all cancers are the same and what works for one person may not work for the next.

Celeste had a dangerous aggressive cancer, Uterine Serous Carcinoma (USC). Chemo treatments worked in the two series of treatments they were administered. No one can say they would not have worked for a third series. A third series would have given Celeste another year, if the treatment worked as it did in the first two series. If the chemo treatments continued to work, each series would have added another year. She was not given the chance. The "experimental" treatments tried by the oncologist killed her. The oncologist's selection of chemicals damaged Celeste's heart and kidneys. I am convinced it was heart failure that took her life away from us so suddenly.

Celeste was within three months of her 94th birthday when the oncologist doctor determined her selection of chemicals was not working and then ordered that there would be no further treatments. Celeste was a young 93 and was sure she would live to be 100. Without the cancer, I strongly believe she would have made it as well.

Chapter 15

CELLULAR FUNCTIONS AND CANCER

It appears that cancer cells originate from a disruption of the cell in some way. The repair mechanism, or simply destruction of the cell and replacing it by a healthy cell, is not functioning. Cancer starts at the cellular level.

One of the first reactions, of the malfunctioning cell, is the production of nitric oxide. When a cell has been injured, nitric oxide and other growth factors are released to signal cells to grow and divide to replace lost cells. In a person with cancer, tumor cells may be in concert with nitric oxide and be signaled to grow. Nitric oxide is known to be a promoter of angiogenesis and tumor progression. A number of other factors are involved in cancer progression. Consider cortisol levels: they are higher in people with cancer. Cortisol in the bloodstream leads to increased production of the hormone estrogen.

A test of memory in a biochemistry class is to be able to diagram what happens in a cell starting with glucose to the production of cellular energy. The steps take one through glycolysis, the Krebs Cycle and Oxidative Phosphorylation to the production of ATP and carbon dioxide.

This is the functioning of a normal cell producing energy by respiration (37.2 billion cells in the human body) using the three steps above. This is known as mitochondrial respiration or oxidative metabolism. This system is highly efficient in producing cellular energy.

A cancerous cell uses glycolysis, the first step, only. The cancer cell ferments the sugar (glucose) and produces lactic acid as a by-product.

This metabolic shift – cellular respiration to glycolysis – occurs because the cell has lost its ability to use oxygen, for reasons not known. Glycolysis does not require oxygen. The Krebs cycle and oxidative phosphorylation do require oxygen but these two phases are not utilized by cancerous cells.

When the cell cannot use oxygen, this is the moment it becomes a cancerous cell, called the Warburg effect. Dr. Otto Warburg, Nobel Prize laureate, in 1930, described a cancer cell as an elevated producer of lactic acid. Lactic acid is known to suppress the immune system, promotes cancer growth and metastasis, and triggers the release of cortisol.

People with the highest cortisol levels, have the greater risk of cancer. There is a blood test for lactic acid, but whether it could be used to detect cancer in the early stages, is not known.

Cortisol in the bloodstream leads to increased production of the hormone estrogen. In the 1990's Women's Health Initiative study tested the effects of supplemental estrogen on women's health. The study was forced to be terminated after participants developed cardiovascular disease, stroke, dementia and cancer.

Daily life is highly stressful. The stress hormone, adrenaline, is a primary trigger for the breakdown of fat. A breakdown of fat includes formation of unsaturated fatty acids, which enter the bloodstream and form prostaglandins, which are carcinogenic.

Cortisol's basic function is to catabolize muscle tissue and muscle meat contains high levels of the amino acid tryptophan (a precursor for serotonin). Stress increases serotonin production. Serotonin represents part of the body's response to stress and has been shown to promote tumor growth.

An elevated blood level of the hormone prolactin, triggers inflammation by amplifying the production of inflammatory cytokines. They promote the formation and progression of numerous types of cancer. Prolactin promotes growth of ovarian surface epithelial cells, inhibits apoptosis and increases survival of ovarian cancer cells. Prolactin is produced in ovaries and may be associated with increased risk of ovarian cancer.

There are a number of other tumor factors that contribute to the microenvironmental of cancers.

One of the most fundamental ways to promote good health is through a healthy diet and activity. A healthy diet addresses the type and quantity of food consumed. Activity promotes both physical and mental health.

Chapter 16
DIET, HEALTH AND CANCER

Cancer starts at the cellular level. When cancer becomes a tumor, it may be too late. If an individual is going to have a say in what is going on within their own body, any action taken must deal with what is happening at the cellular level.

Cancer fighting foods should be a way of life to minimize risk of being diagnosed with cancer. The following list of foods does not include all of the foods which may be beneficial in warding off a diagnosis of cancer, but it is a start.

Foods alone cannot contain or cure cancer, but nutrition plays a large role in supporting the immune system. The gut controls the body and an individual must control what gets into the gut. To a large extent, each make choices of the food consumed. Eating healthy appeals to many and the opposite is also true. Obesity and ill health, in many cases, are the result of lifetime choices. Diet resistant obesity, is the new victim status.

Let's get started with good food choices. Apples contain polyphenols, plant-based compounds that prevent inflammation, cardiovascular disease, and infections. The polyphenol phloretin inhibits a protein glucose transporter 2(GLUT2) which has a role in advanced-stage cell growth in certain types of cancer.

Berries are rich in vitamins, minerals, and dietary fiber; the brighter the color the more beneficial. The berry contains phytochemicals called anthocyanins. They are known to stop new blood vessels from forming to prevent cancer cells from obtaining oxygen. Berries are packed with antioxidants that attack free radicals that damage cell membranes.

Broccoli, cauliflower and kale contain beneficial nutrients as vitamin C, vitamin K and manganese. Cruciferous vegetables contain sulforaphane, a plant compound with anticancer properties.

Carrots contain vitamins A, K, antioxidants, and beta-carotene, responsible for the orange color. Beta-carotene supports the immune system.

All nuts possess anti-cancer properties. Walnuts contain a substance called pedunculagin, which is metabolized to form urolithins, compounds that bind estrogen receptors. The involvement of estrogen in cancer formation continually surfaces.

Beans, peas, and lentils, are high in fiber and protein. Black and Navy beans, particularly, have high levels of the fatty acid butyrate, they have a low glycemic index which prevents blood-sugar levels from spiking.

Tomatoes are a brightly colored food, highly beneficial for endometrial, lung, prostate, and stomach cancers; high in antitoxins, viable tool for flushing out cancer-inducing toxins from the body. They are an excellent source of dietary lycopene, the carotenoid responsible for the red color. They were first brought from South America to Europe.

Garlic is rich in vitamin C, vitamin B6, thiamin, potassium, calcium, phosphorus, copper and manganese. Onions are a good source of vitamin C, vitamin B6, potassium and folate. Onions and garlic add flavor to foods without resorting to butter and salt. Garlic and onions along with shallots, leeks and chives; are of the allium family. These foods are often considered medicinal foods. Allium vegetables are rich in organosulfur compounds which may be beneficial for lowering cholesterol and blood pressure while helping to prevent chronic conditions including cancer and cardiovascular disease.

Turmeric is a yellow-orange powder form from the root of the plant. The active ingredient is curcumin, a powerful ingredient in an anti-cancer diet. It has been known to shrink tumor size, especially in colon and breast cancer. It contains high levels of capsicum (chili powder).

Carotenoid antioxidants are found in fruits and vegetables. Pumpkin, squash, sweet potatoes, oranges, nectarines, and more. The particular carotenoids found in these foods are alpha-carotene, beta-carotene, lycopene, cryptoxanthin. They also contain lutein and zeaxanthin.

Healthy fatty acids account for 60 percent of brain and the nervous system. Healthy fatty acids include oils as flaxseed oil, coconut oil, palm oil, cod liver oil, and extra virgin olive oil. These unrefined oils promote digestion and raise immunity level.

Apple cider vinegar is a natural source of fermented goodness and one of the primary cure-alls known to man.

Leafy green vegetables are eminently enhancing and disease fighting. They are high in minerals, vitamins and key nutrients. They are low in calories, fat, sodium, additives and supply key nutrients. This includes spinach, romaine lettuce, cabbage, kale, and flat-leafed vegetables. They also contain high levels of vitamin C and beta-carotene. They contain anti-bacterial and anti-viral properties.

The discussion of unsaturated and saturated fats gets much attention, especially as regards heart health. Coconut oil is a 93 percent saturated fat, 4 percent monounsaturated fat and 3 percent unsaturated fat. Coconut oil is a stable medium chain length triglyceride and seemingly is readily digested. Unsaturated fats include oils that are liquid at room temperature as corn, soy, canola, hemp, flax, sunflower, safflower, peanut and fish oil. The unsaturated fats oxidize readily and are unstable.

Coconut is a fruit, a seed and a nut that grows on palm trees in over 90 countries worldwide. Its meat, juice, milk and oil have been staples in the diets of many cultures for generations.

The word coconut is derived from the 16th century Portuguese and Spanish word coco, meaning "head" or "skull", as the three indentations on its hairy shell resemble a face. Due to its high level of saturated fats, coconut oil is stable and protected from reacting with oxygen and become oxidized. Coconut oil has been stored up to a year at room temperature without becoming rancid. A Columbia University scientist wrote in 1992 that it was safest to use in cooking. Unsaturated fats are unsaturated fatty acids and are highly unstable and react readily with oxygen to form multiple reaction products.

All available population studies show dietary coconut oil does not lead to high serum cholesterol nor to high coronary heart disease mortality.

Atherosclerotic plaques readily incorporate n-3 (omega-3) from fish-oil supplements and lead to linear increase in arterial plaque with continued consumption. Men advised to eat oily fish, and particularly those supplemented with fish oil capsules, had a higher risk of cardiac death.

Saturated fats have long been blamed for "heart disease" yet there are no scientific studies that prove there is a link between saturated fat intake and cardiovascular disease.

A 1978 study of the people of Sri Lankan who consumed a high rate of coconut oil as the main dietary fat had the lowest death rate from heart disease in the world. Population studies show that dietary coconut oil does not lead to high serum cholesterol or coronary heart disease mortality.

Island-dwelling Polynesian populations near the equator known as Pukapuka derive 63 Percent of their nutrition from coconut. A 1981 study revealed that their rates of cardiovascular disease were nearly non-existant.

Dr. Aseem Malkhotra, Cardiologist at the Croydon University Hospital in London, England wrote in 2013, "The mantra that saturated fat must be removed to reduce the risk of cardiovascular disease has dominated dietary advice and guidelines for almost four decades. Yet scientific evidence shows that this advice has, paradoxically, increased our cardiovascular risks."

A study published in the *British Medical Journal,* concluded, "Saturated fats are not associated with all-cause mortality, cardiovascular disease, coronary heart disease, stroke, or type 2 diabetes…" Dietary saturated fats protect the heart and reduce the risk of cardiovascular disease.

Since 1945 it has been hypothesized that unsaturated fats enhance tumors and that saturated fats as coconut oil, protect against tumor formation. Research has demonstrated that tumor-induced animals fed the least amount of unsaturated fats had the least tumors.

A 2016 study found an inverse relationship between saturated fat and tumor burden in rats. High saturated fat was protective and a decrease in mortality in mice consuming the highest concentration of saturated fatty acids.

Looking at cancer preventative diets, it appears the lower the unsaturated fat intake the better.

Healthy life styles, healthy foods and healthy genetics generally are an excellent combination that leads to longevity. People living in Azerbaijan are noted for being long-lived. A study of staple food in the diet, revealed that fresh fruit and vegetables made up a large part of the diet.

Fatty meats are tasty but they may not be the best foods for longevity and weight control. That single factor of consideration has resulted in high intake of meats as chicken and turkey.

References:

1. Ridgeway, S. (2016). Different Uses for a Coconut. https://caloriebee. com/nutrition/Differnt -Uses-for-a Coconut.
2. Debmandal M, Mandal S. Coconut (Cocos nucifera L.: Arecaceae: in health promotion and disease prevention. *Asian Pac J Trop Med.* 2011;4(3):241-7.
3. Delgado, S.R. 1982. Glossario Iuso-asiatico, Part 1. Buske Verlag.
4. Morgradean D, Poiana MA, Gogoasa I. Quality characteristics and oxidative stability of coconut oil during storage. *J Agro. Proc. & Tech* 2012;18(4):272-276.
5. Kaunitz H. Coconut oil consumption and coronary heart disease. *Agris.* 1992.
6. Marina AM, et al. Chemical properties of virgin coconut oil. *J. Amer. Oil. Chem. Soc.* 2009;86(4):301-307.
7. Rapp JH, et al. Dietary eicosapentaenoic acid and docosahexaeoic acid from fish oil. Their incorporation into advanced human atherosclerotic plaques. *Artderioscler Thromb.* 1991;11(4):903-11.
8. Burr ML, Ashfield-watt PA, Dunstan FD, et al. Lack of benefitd of dietary advice to men with angina: results f a controlled trial. *Eur J Clin Nutr.* 2003;57(2):193-200.
9. Siri-tarino PW, Sun Q, Hu FB, Krauss RM. Meta-analysis of prospective cohort studies evaluating the association of saturated fat with cardiovascular disease. *Am J Clin Nutr.* 201;91(3):535-46.
10. Kaunitz H. Medium chain triglycerides (MCT) in aging and arteriosclerosis. *J Environ Pathol Toxicol Oncol.* 1986;6(3-4):115-21.
11. Prior IA, et al. Cholesterol, coconuts, and diet on Polynesian atolls: a natural experiment: the Pukapuka and Tokelau island studies. Am J Clin Nutr. 1981;34(8):1552-61.
12. Malhotra A. Saturated fat is not the major issue. *BMJ.* 2013;347:f6340.
13. De souza RJ, et al. Intake of saturated and trans unsaturated fatty acids and risk ofd all cause mortality, cardiovascular disease, and type 2 diabetes: systematic review and meta-analysis of observational studies. *BMJ.* 2005;351:h3978.

14. Mozaffarian D, Rimm EBF, Herrington DMH. Dietary fats, carbohydrate, and progression of coronary atherosclerosis in postmenopausal women. *Am J Clin Nutr.* 2004;80(5):1175-84.

15. Cohen, LA. Fat and endocrine-responsive cancer in animals. *Prev Med.* 1987;16(4):468-74.

16. Enos, RT, et al. High-fat diets rich in saturated fat protect against azoxymethane/dextran sulfate sodium induced colon cancer. *Am J Physiol Gastrointest Liver Physiol.* 2016;310(11): G906-19.

Chapter 17

REFLECTIONS

Having lost a wonderful person to the curse of ovarian cancer, I have reflections about many things.

First, I am convinced that Celeste contracted ovarian cancer as a result of consumption of a large quantity of milk over her lifetime. With that thought in mind, for the last 10 years she reduced her milk intake to one eight-ounce glass per day. The high rate of milk consumption over the previous 80-year period and the continued consumption of milk every day over the last ten years, loaded her system with estrogen and galactose. The damage caused by both, along with all of the contaminants in milk and dairy products; she ended up with the worst variant of ovarian cancer, Uterus Serous Carcinoma. This I firmly believe.

The 1990's Women's Health Initiative study tested the effects of supplemental estrogen on women, but was forced to stop because participants began developing cardiovascular disease, stroke, dementia and cancer. (2). Was this a warning about estrogen in milk? Should something have been done about what happened? Should all of the news media have jumped on it to warn people about the hazards of estrogen in milk?

I have given considerable thought to how fast cancer develops as well. Earlier, I indicated that it takes an average of 6.5 years for cancer cells to travel from the fallopian tubes to the ovary. Then how many decades does it take to convert a normal cell to a cancerous cell and then form a tumor? Earlier it was mentioned that it takes up to 60 mutations to develop a cancerous cell. Then how long is it until a tumor is noticed? When a tumor as ovarian cancer forms, there is nothing restricting the cells from sloughing off and floating to anywhere in the uninhibited chamber

As I reviewed milk, the politics, the potential contamination, the injection of hormones in the cows, antibiotics for mammary glands and udder infections (mastitis), the level of somatic cells allowed in milk, the galactose sugar from milk; all add up to one thing. If Celeste had not consumed milk and dairy products, I cannot help but think she would still be with us and enjoying life to the fullest.

Today, 2022, there is no need for cow's milk in the diet. It is too great a risk to take. Milk and milk products are not needed in the nutrition of humans any more than milk and dairy products are needed for the nutrition of chickens, hogs, cows, horses or sheep and goats.

Heart disease, high cholesterol, along with high blood pressure, many types of cancer and the politics associated with dairy, cost to taxpayers etc. all add up, in my mind, to an overwhelming denial of milk and dairy products.

There is almond, coconut, oat, soy, rice, and perhaps many more kinds of milk, if a milk is required for any reason. All would be healthier, there would not be a health concern, no one would have to worry about the contamination, the politics, governmental subsidies, and the irritation of the continued promotion and illusions of a healthy product needed for all. I personally have not consumed milk for over 70 years and eat only limited quantities of dairy products that are in prepared foods. I consider myself much healthier because of my denial of milk and milk products.

Where is the progress on solving the awful disease of ovarian cancer? Since 1971, $500 billion dollars have been spent on cancer research (1). The American Cancer Society has been the place to get big grant money. Most every research organization, has a staff of grant writers. Universities are at the head of this group. They know the language and the "secrets" to write grant proposals that entice large grants for "research". Each does a literature review and puts together a proposal and submits it with "professionalism." When sitting on a huge pile of money, the granter doles out to "researchers" who prepare the best sounding sell job. A publishable paper is a requirement. These papers are "peer" reviewed. At Universities the "research" is generally conducted by a graduate student. The major professor supervising the research has gained much expertise at writing proposals and may have any number of graduate students and they "crank out" the papers. The peers all use the same language. When the paper is written it will be full of could, may, might, etc. Each paper is much the same by the same researchers and each tries to add a little something in order to get the next huge grant. This has been going on for the last 50 years or more and the progress has been atrocious.

This "cancer research" piles up in the libraries. That is not where it is needed. A lot of good people must take the information from the library to the clinic and solve this horrific disease.

The progress of ovarian cancer is only one example. When a new cancer patient is recruited, the outline of the treatment is surgery and chemo. Chemo has been around for 50 years and the chemicals used today are 30 years in existence. Surgery has been around for over a 100-years and it gets more complicated for the patient yearly. In advanced cancer cases, so much of the body is removed, it is a wonder the patient survives. Then the chemical treatments are so harsh that the patient dies from the treatment after destruction of vital organs as heart, liver and kidneys. Yes, there are survivors past five years, but they have paid a price.

We have seen how the American Cancer Society (ACS), The Food and Drug Administration (FDA), the American Dairy Association (ADA), and Monsanto stuck together attacking Dr. Epstein's article in the Los Angeles Times earlier. Few scientists can match the career record of Dr. Epstein. They will attack anyone who dares to speak out.

What would happen if there was no cancer and no milk? How would all of these people survive? What would happen to all of these people who now have a livelihood off of both of these enterprises? Remember that there are a lot of attorneys involved with these organizations and a lot of doctors holding administrative positions.

Is a lot of all of this research a farce? Is there a certain amount of dishonesty in turning out article after article and overloading libraries and in the end coming up with close to nothing in the way of "progress"?

In the words of Dr. Glen Warner, "We have a multi-billion-dollar industry that is killing people, right and left, just for financial gain." Celeste was one of these. She was treated with technology over 40 years old and the two drugs that were used have been patented and cleared by the FDA for nearly 30 years. But they worked, but then the cancer doctor in charge changed the treatment to known destructive chemicals that damaged her heart and kidneys, why? This doctor considers herself autonomous and she did not feel that she had to explain anything to us. She so reminded me of the following episode.

There was the story of the automobile mechanic who worked on a doctor's car. The doctor complained that the mechanic did not fix his car right. The mechanic replied, that is the difference between me and you, you as a doctor can bury your mistakes. That is how I feel about the cancer doctor that was responsible for the treatment of Celeste!

We receive such praise as to how the cancer treatments "save" lives. I knew a surgeon who was retired who stated, "When I was practicing as a surgeon, whenever someone came in with a problem, I would just cut it out." That is how cancer is looked at today. In many cases, the surgery is massive and how an induvial survives is a marvel. Then as soon as possible, their bodies are ravaged with chemotherapy. It is a wonder anyone survives (and maybe they really don't, we are told they do!). This description of cancer treatment has not changed in 50 years. The lack of cancer diagnostic tests should be considered a public health disaster. Cancer can be resolved only if diagnosed in the early stages (I am beginning to wonder if even this is true). There is no diagnostic test for early detection of ovarian cancer.

It is beginning to appear that the real chance we have to prevent cancer is to defeat it at the cellular level. You ask, how can this be done? The chapter on antioxidants, is a start.

The numerous articles on food are gaining more avid followers. The ingredients in many foods have been identified as promoting good health and they should be a part of a healthy diet. High concentration of these workable food extracts is likely where real progress will come. Vitamin C is a notable example and it should catch the attention of all.

Consider flavonoids, naturally occurring substances found in colorful fruits, vegetables, teas and wines. Epidemiological studies have shown reduction in a number of health problems by consumption of flavonoids. More than 60 flavonoids have been identified in citrus fruit. Flavonoids are more plentiful in the peel than in the fruit itself. Start with eating the peel of a small orange, the mandarin.

Examples of flavonoids in citrus are: naringin, naringenin, diosmin, hesperetin, hesperidin, quercetin, tangeretin, and nobiletin. The potential of using these extractions in a concentrated form may provide a great cancer patient future.

Testing of drugs or nutrients against cancer in a test tube is called *in vitro*. Testing in the body is called *in vivo*. In vitro studies have confirmed naringin inhibits the growth of many kinds of cancer cells.

In vivo studies in animals, when carcinogenic chemicals are injected, naringin inhibited growth of several types of cancer. (3)

A Chinese study tested naringin in 2016 on skin cancer cells. Cancer cells produce lactic acid but naringin inhibited production of lactic acid. They concluded naringin inhibited the malignant phenotype of A375 cells. (4)

Naringenin was also studied in vitro and found to inhibit the growth of a number of cancer cells. A synergistic effect of naringenin was found when combined with curcumin or vitamin E.

Hesperidin was noted to inhibit growth of various cancers in vitro as well.

Oranges have been noted to reduce essentially all of the known products in the cancer tumor as cortisol, nitric oxide, lactic acid, estrogen, prostaglandins, etc.

This discussion helps to bring attention to the beneficial results from citrus in the diet, especially oranges. The helpful role of vitamin C cannot be overstressed.

Vitamin C, ascorbic acid or ascorbate, was officially discovered in 1928 by Hungarian biochemist Albert Szent-Gyorgyi. The first manifestations of vitamin C deficiency were documented by the physician Hippocrates in ancient Greece (460-370 BC).

Vitamin C supplemental doses are highly dependent upon the amount administered. In low doses, vitamin C behaves as an antioxidant, enabling the body to neutralize toxins and eliminate waste products. At high concentrations, vitamin C acts as a prooxidant, selectively targeting unhealthy and even cancerous cells. (11). High-doses of intravenous vitamin C have been used for cancer therapy since the 1970s (5).

Cancer patients have significantly depleted levels of vitamin C. (6) Some researchers believe vitamin C may be the most important nutrient needed by the body to resist cancer cells. (7) Vitamin C in conjunction with B12 can synergistically enhance apoptosis in multiple types of cancer cells. (8)

Vitamin C has been shown to prevent the growth of a number of cancers in animal studies as well. (9)

Linus Pauling, was a two-time Nobel Prize winner in clay mineralogy (Pauling's rules) and for his work with vitamin C. He and chief surgeon Ewan Cameron of Vale of Leven Hospital in Scotland, as early as 1976, demonstrated that 10 grams per day of vitamin C increased the survival rate of terminal cancer patients 4.2 times compared to patients receiving no vitamin C. Life was extended up to six years with vitamin C compared to 6 months without vitamin C. (6)

It is believed when blood levels are maintained at a consistently high level of vitamin C, the vitamin C is absorbed into cancerous tissue, producing hydrogen peroxide which actually kills cancer cells. (10) In high doses, vitamin C acts as a pro-oxidant that can selectively target unhealthy and even cancerous cells. (11)

A 2008 study at the National Institutes of Health reported high-doses of vitamin C resulted in cytotoxicity of a variety of cancer cells invitro without adversely affecting normal cells. (9)

Dr. Frederick R. Klenner demonstrated 70 years ago that vitamin C doses as high as 300 grams per day (300,000mg) in humans are safe and modern research has confirmed it. (12)

High levels of ascorbic acid (vitamin C) can increase the absorption of iron which may become toxic in excess. (13) Oral supplements might be best administered without food. Iron chelating substances as tetracycline or curcumin may be helpful. (14)

Blood levels of vitamin C have been reported as high as 400 microM/L (moles per liter) with liposomal vitamin C. (15) Vitamin C blood levels of 250 microM/L have been achieved with a single 5-gram oral dose of vitamin C. (15)

Maximum blood levels of vitamin C may be achieved by consuming approximately 3 grams vitamin C every four hours. Vitamin C is only active in the body for a few hours so frequent doses must be administered to maintain consistently high blood levels. (16)

Chemotherapy often will damage the kidneys and liver. Vitamin C has been shown to prevent this damage. (17)

Lactic acid is produced by cells that are not getting what they need to produce energy efficiently. Lactic acid suppresses the immune system (18), promotes cancer growth and metastasis (19). Vitamin C prevents the formation of nitric oxide. (20) Consumption of oranges can reduce nitric oxide (21). Does anyone test for lactic acid? It is a normal part of a blood test but it must be requested. Can nitric oxide be determined in a blood test?

People with cancer have higher cortisol levels than people without cancer (22). Oranges reduce cortisol levels (23) and any number of tumor microenvironment elements.

The food one consumes is used to power the energy-producing system within each of the cells, called mitochondria. One of the most fundamental ways to aid human health in a positive way is to consume foods that are nutritious and known to support good health.

Prolactin – Elevated blood concentrations of hormone prolactin trigger inflammation by amplifying the production of inflammatory cytokines, and promote the formation and progression of numerous types of cancer. Prolactin promotes growth of ovarian surface epithelial cells and inhibits apoptosis and increases survival of ovarian cancer cells. Prolactin is produced in the pituitary gland and in ovaries and other areas of the body. How can it be controlled?

Cortisol-People with cancer have higher levels of cortisol than normal. Cancer patients with the highest level of Cortisol have the greatest risk of dying from the disease. (24)

The presence of cortisol in the bloodstream leads to increased production of the hormone estrogen. The Women's Health Initiative in the 1990s testing the effect of supplemental estrogen had to be cancelled because of ill effects.

Serotonin- The basic action of serotonin is to catabolize muscle tissue. After sugar in the blood cells has been diminished, cancer cells attack muscle tissue. About ninety percent of advanced cancer patients are affected by anorexia and muscle wasting (cachexia). (25) Muscle contains high levels of the amino acid tryptophan (a precursor for serotonin) Stress increases serotonin production amplifying the production of cytokines and promote the formation and progression of numerous types of cancer.

Routine tests to monitor cortisol, estrogen, serotonin, histamine, nitric oxide, lactic acid, prolactin, etc. might lead to early diagnosis.

Histamine is an inflammatory mediator known for its role in allergic reactions. Substances that inhibit histamine have been observed to prevent cancer growth and progression.

Scientist test the therapeutic value of nutrients or drugs against cancer by adding substances to a test tube containing cancer cells and observe the results.

Flavonoids are naturally occurring substances found in fruits, vegetables, teas and wines responsible for a diversity of colors produced by plants. Studies have shown that consumption of flavonoids can reduce the risk of several diseases and health problems.

More than 60 flavonoids have been identified in citrus fruit. Flavonoids are more abundant in the peel than in the pulp of citrus fruit.

When a natural substance is found in foods, it cannot be patented or sold by drug companies. This type of research is not often funded and the research is rarely performed. Often, the only reason in vitro and in vivo studies on food nutrients are funded is so drug companies can find components that work and then attempt to replicate similar chemicals to patent and sell. The cost of in vitro and in vivo to test humans in a clinical testing trial phase 1 in the U.S. may cost millions of dollars. Then the cost for this new chemical may be prohibitive.

References:

1. The American Cancer Society.com
2. Sloan, Mark. (2018) Cancer: The Metabolic Disease Unravelled. ENDALLDISEASE Publishing. ISBN:978-0-99-47418-5-1. p.3
3. Sloan, Mark. Ibid. p-17
4. Guo B, Zhang Y, Hui Q, Wang H, Tao K. Naringin suppresses the metabolism of A375 cells y inhibiting the phosphorylation of the c-Src. *Tumor Biol*. 2016;37(3):3841-50.
5. Venturelli S, Sinnberg TW, Niessner H, Busch C. Moledular mehanisms of pharmacological doses of ascorbate on cancer cells. Wien, *Med Wochenschr*. 2015;165(11-12):251-7.

6. Cameron E, Pauling L. Supplemental ascorbate in the supportive treatment of cancer: Prolongation of survival times in terminal human cancer. *Proc Natl Acad* Sci USA. 1976;73(10):3685-9.

7. Cameron E. Vitamin C and cancer: an overview. *Int J Vitam Nur Res Bad Phosphorylation*. 1982;23:115-27.

8. Chen N, Yin S, Song X, Fan L, Hu H. Vitamin B2 Sensitizes Cancer Cells to Vitamin-C-Induced Cell Death via Modulation of Akt and Bad Phosphorylation. *J Agri Foods Chem*. 2015;63(30):6739-48.

9. Chen Q, Espewy MG, Sun AY, et al. Pharmacologic doses of ascorbate act as a prooxidant and decrease growth of aggressive tumor xenografts in mice. *Proc Natl Acad Sci USA*. 12008;105(32):11105-9.

10. PDQ Cancer Information Sumaries- High-dose Vitamin C. 2015. http://www.ncbi.nlm.nih.gov/books/NBK127724/#CDR00000752253.

11. Mastrangelo D, Massai L, Lo coco F, et al. Cytotoxic effects of high concentrations of sodium ascorbate on human myeloid cell lines. Ann Hematol. 2015;94(ll):1807-16.

12. Gonzalez MJ, Miranda-massare JR, Berdiel MJ, et al. High Dose Intraveneous Vitamin C and Chikungunya Fever: . F A Case Report. *J. Orthomol, Med*. 2014;29(4):154-156

13. Lane, DJ, Richardson DR. The active role of vitamin C in mammalian iron metabolism: much more than just enhanced iron absorption! Free *Radic Biol Med*. 2014;75:69-83.

14. Jiao Y, Wilkinson J, Di X, et al. Curcumin, a cancer chemopreventive and chemotherapeutic agent, is a biological active iron chelator. Blood. 2009;113(2):462-9.

15. Hickey, S., & Saul, A.W. (2008), *Vitamin C: The real story: The remarkable and controversial healing factor*. Laguna Beach, CA: Basic Health Publications.

16. Sloan, Mark. (20-18) Cancer, The Metabolic Disease Unravelled. ENDALLDISEASE Publishing. ISBN:978-0-9947418-5-1.p-3.

17. Chen MF, Yang CMm Au XMm GU ML Vitamin C protects against cisplatin-induce nephrotoxicity and damage without reducing its effectiveness inC57BL/6 mice xenografted with Lewis lung carcinoma. *Nutr Cancer*. 2014;66(7):1085-91.

18. Bodduluru LN, Kasala ER, Madhana RM, et al. Naringenin ameliorates inflammation and cell proliferation in benzo(a)pyrene

induced pulmonary carcinogenesis by modulating CYP1A1, NFxB and PCNA epression. *Int Immunopharmacol.* 2016;30:102-10

19. Sabarinathan D, Mahakalakshmi P, Vanisree AJ. Naringenin promote apoptosis in cerebrally implanted C6 glioma cells. *Mol Cell Biochem.* 2010;345(1-2):215-22.

20. Mckinnon RL, Lidington D, Tyml K. Ascorbate inhibits reduced arteriolar conducted vasoconstriction in septic mouse cremaster muscle. Microcirculation. 2007;14(7):697-707.Xu T, 21. Wang L, Tao Y, Ji Y, Deng F, Wu XH. The function of Naringin in Inducing Secretion of Osteoprotegerin and Inhibiting Formation of Osteoclasts. Evid Based Complement *Altermat Med.* 2016;2016:89811650

21. Casey SC, Amedei Ad, Aquilano K, et al. Cancere prevetion and therapy through the modulation of the tumor microenvironment Semin Cancer Biol. 2015;35Suppl:S199-223.

22. Kawaguchi K, Maruyama H, Hasunuma R, Kumazawa Y. Suppression of inflammatory responses after onset of collagen-induced arthritis in mice by oral administration of the Citrus flavanone naringin. *Immunopharmacol Immunotoxicol.* 2011:33(4):723-9.

23. Sun Y, Gu J. Study on effect of naringenin in inhibiting migration and invasion of breast cancer cells and its molecular mechanism. Zhongguo Zhong Yao Za Zhi. 201;40(6):1144-50.

24. Cheng LI, Liu YY, Li B, Li SY Ran PX. An in vitro study on the pharmacological ascorbate treatment of influenza virus. *Zhonghua Jie He He Hu Xi Za Zhi.* 2012;35(7):520-30.

Chapter 18

CLOSING THOUGHTS

The opinion I have of the doctor who had the responsibility of care of Celeste's treatments is that I will never allow this doctor to ever have a say in any medical opinion in the future.

The first occasion I had to have an ill opinion of this doctor was after the first series of chemo treatment, she told us that "the cancer was gone." Celeste was diagnosed with Uterine Serous Carcinoma, Stage III. This is a cancer that accounts for 10 percent of all endometrial cancers. But this cancer accounts for 80 percent of all endometrial cancer related deaths. Any doctor who had ever treated this cancer previously would have known how utterly tragic this cancer is and yet she uttered such a foolish egregious statement.

Not once did this doctor mention the type of cancer Celeste had nor ever infer the seriousness of the cancer.

Then she decided to perform robotic surgery when she said Celeste only had dead tissue and scar tissue. The person administering the anesthesia for the surgery charged $2300 under a code that neither Medicare nor Tri Care could pay, "extreme age". In other words, it was an extra $2300 charge. I assume this person was a cohort of hers and these extra charges were routine. The "surgery" lasted less than an hour, from start to finish.

The two series of chemo were routine using technology that was 30 years old. Both chemicals, Carboplatin and Paclitaxel (Taxol), were approved for chemo in the early nineties. The most precise part involved preparing the chemicals prior to injection to ensure dose measured up to weight, etc.

After completion of the last of the second series, the doctor stated that Celeste could have the portal removed that was used for injection of the chemo treatments (meaning no more chemo treatments).

Perhaps this would have been the time to ask some penetrating questions. Celeste was now 93 years old. She had been able to handle the chemo treatments well and led a near normal life. She maintained her usual weight, her skin color was good, she actively worked out at the gym and water aerobic classes. She was at the gym five days weekly unless absence was required because of doctor appointments. Celest never experienced nausea while on the chemo treatments. She was actively engaged in caring for her plants. In early November she had the electric hedge trimmer fine tuning the trimming of her globe edge plants.

After completion of the second series of chemo treatments, the CA-125 cancer antibody blood test registered 29.6 on February 24, 2021. This is in the "normal" range.

The next CA-125 test administered on July 27, 2021, six months later, was 363.1. This was the highest number to date. Why the doctor in charge of Celeste waited nearly six months to allow the cancer to rebuild so high will never be answered.

The chemo treatments had both been highly successful in lowering the CA-125 blood test, and I can only assume that meant the cancer was controlled. Celeste was able to tolerate the chemo and she was doing well. In any other endeavor, with this kind of success, "you go with them that 'brung' you here." The chemo treatments worked and should have been continued.

This doctor decided, on her own, to yank something off the shelf that has been used by other doctors. I have no idea if she ever had any experience with the drug, but it was a horrific choice.

The drug she selected was "a biosimilar biologic medical product that is almost an identical copy of an original medication that is manufactured by a different pharmaceutical company." This biosimilar drug was: Mvasi. It was supposedly biosimilar to Bevacizumab, trade name: Avastin. It is not a chemo drug but a "monoclonal antibody" and "anti-angiogenesis" drug. This was a complete switch from a known treatment regime to a completely unknown. The patient is at the mercy of the "doctor". With each day, the cancer cells were exploding and yet there was no urgency on the part of the doctor. After all, she only spent one day every two weeks to tend to patients.

The first treatment of the "biosimilar" drug was given on June 14. The final chemo treatment was given on January 6, 2021. The CA-125 blood test on February 24, 2021 was 29.6, in the "normal" range. Five months passed when no treatments were given. In the meantime, the CA 125 was not monitored as well. The second and third treatments of the "biosimilar" drug were given July 6 and July 27. By July 27, the CA-125 blood test had reached 363.l, indicating that this new chemical had no effect in lowering the cancer antigen number. Celeste was experiencing Nephrotic Syndrome, high levels of protein in the urine, indicating kidney damage.

The next "experimental" drug to be tried by this doctor was Gemcitabine or Gemzar but not until September 17. On July 27, it was known that the CA 125 was at 363.1 (0-30 normal). This doctor did nothing for two months. Two additional treatments were given on October 19 and October 27. No CA-125 blood tests were taken until October 18 when the CA-125 blood test had rocketed to 695.

To put this picture in perspective, the last chemo treatment was given on January 6. Nothing was done for five months plus one week. The chemo treatments, based on the CA-125 blood test, worked wonders as confirmed by the February 24, 2021, test of 29.6. Because of the five-month delay, the cancer has accelerated to an all-time high of 363.1 and there was no monitoring of the CA-125 blood test.

Then three treatments of a non-chemo chemical damaged the kidneys and was stopped on July 27. It had no effect on the CA-125.

Then nothing was done from July 27 until September 17, when the next new chemical treatment started. Two additional treatments were given.

The potassium spiked for the first time on October 13 resulting in a three-day hospital stay October 14-16 to stabilize the blood potassium. Celeste was experiencing Nephrotic Syndrome, high levels of protein in the urine, indicating kidney damage. She spent time in the hospital on three different occasions in an effort to stabilize the potassium level in her blood.

Then came the appointment with the cancer doctor on November 10. This doctor was in the office one day every two weeks. Her regular office was 100 miles away. It appears she either lost interest in having Celeste as a patient or her incompetence surfaced, or both, as she fumbled with what to do next. The choice to continue the same chemo treatments that worked would have been an easy and the right decision.

This doctor never spent five minutes with any appointment we ever had with her. She never discussed any tests. She did not feel that she had to discuss anything about this case with us. The fateful decision on November 10 was no exception. She came in, sat down on her stool, and said since nothing was working, Celeste would be turned over to hospice (to die.) End of visit!

Celeste looked straight into the eyes of the doctor and said nothing. I looked at Celeste and what I saw was a lovely lady who looked like she always did. Her weight was her normal weight. She looked healthy; she was doing everything she had done in the past. She had life, she was alive! If she had stayed on chemo, I have no idea how long she might have still been with us. Instead, here was a doctor ordering her execution.

Celeste was not a helpless cancer eaten skin and bones victim unable to hold her head up in a wheel chair. She had just returned from one of her favorite places in the world, South Padre Island, where she charged the water breakers as a teenager. She was full of life. She undertook the cancer treatments to live. And now this doctor was telling her to go home and let the cancer grow until it kills her. This is how we treat cancer in the U.S.? Despicable! (or much worse!)

We always consider that the doctor knows best. In this case, this doctor did not know what was best. Her announcement was brutal, heartless, lacked compassion and sympathy, cruel, cold-blooded, callous, insensitive or any of a dozen other terms to vividly describe her action. If anyone asked me about her professionalism in the future, I would say, get as far away from her as possible, as fast as possible!

Chapter 19

SUMMARY OF THE CANCER EXPERIENCE

Get your facts first, then you can distort them as you please.

----Mark Twain

I am now the same age Celeste was when she was first diagnosed with cancer. I am putting myself in her position and I am thinking how I would react to being diagnosed with a killer cancer now that I have gone through the treatment process available for cancer patients.

Celeste was diagnosed by the family physician after the medical staff went through the usual diagnostic tools available. Basically, the decision naming the type of cancer was verified by the CT scan and a biopsy. The cancer cells from the biopsy are stained and examined under a microscope. The cancer is identified by the color and shape of the cancer cells.

The cancer was identified as Uterine Papillary Serous Carcinoma. Uterine Serous Carcinoma (USC) is a very similar kind of cancer. The cancer was in stage III. It was known from the get-go that the cancer was a highly malignant form of endometrial adenocarcinoma. It is a clinically aggressive and a morphological distinct variant and spreads more quickly than other common forms of endometrial cancer. It was identified as a type II cancer, which is immune to hormone treatment. Type II cancers have other differences from type I cancers as well. Perhaps the most notable feature is the death ratio of type II cancers is much higher. As was stated earlier in the text, the uterine papillary serous carcinoma accounts for less than 10% of all endometrial cancers and 80% of endometrial cancer related deaths.

The family doctor knew the seriousness of the cancer and knew that any prognosis would be bad, although he did not discuss a prognosis. What he did say in the same interview was that "palliative" care would be an option. Palliative care is little different from Hospice. Palliative care is comfort care with or without curative intent. Hospice is comfort care without curative intent.

Perhaps a more definitive difference between the two treatments is that Hospice care costs are paid 100 percent by Medicare. Palliative costs can vary. The patient must understand this difference and utilize insurance plans, copay and other measures but must fully understand the cost to the patient in advance.

No one discussed prognosis" at any time. No one ever mentioned the term "terminal". No one ever stated that this is a dangerous cancer. People in the cancer business are close-vested. By that, I mean they say "nothing". They tell what treatments are to be given, period! They never discussed the CT or PET scans, blood tests except to say the white and red blood cells showed up low on the blood test.

After the first series of 12 chemo treatments, the doctor with supervision over Celeste's case told us, "The cancer is gone"! This was a falsehood and no one could imagine another doctor making such an inane statement. Anyone who has ever witnessed one case of this type cancer would know that there are likely no survivors of this cancer. Based on this statement and what transpired later, any statement I could make about this doctor would be excessively generous.

I must place myself in the center of the circumstance that Celeste faced when being informed that she had cancer. The type of cancer was only additional information at the time. I don't believe we even considered how dangerous the cancer might be. After all, the bombshell that one has been struck with cancer is all inclusive. Secondly, the only thought Celeste had at the time was the cancer treatments would allow her to live and continue to enjoy life.

I learned that the median for her cancer is 40 months for those who take cancer treatments. That means, 50% of the patients will die before 40 months. Half will live longer. Celeste lived less time than half of the patients, 30 months. For those who choose not to take cancer treatments, I cannot say what the time outcome might be and I am certain no one in the cancer business would ever hazard a guess. Celeste fully expected that she would be one of the long survivors because of her otherwise good health, physical condition, weight control, gym activities and determination. The oncology doctor calling the shots determined Celeste's early demise.

Celeste essentially continued her normal activities during the time she was undertaking chemo therapy. She was able to tolerate the chemo treatments. COVID-19 soon came on the scene and that forced a limit on activities. The Monday bridge sessions were terminated due to COVID. She so enjoyed the challenge of the bridge game and missed the friends and acquaintances. At the same time, the threat of COVID prevented taking cruises. Actually, any grouping of people was discouraged. She so loved South Padre Island and COVID, along with cancer treatments, reduced opportunities to enjoy the beach and the water. She especially enjoyed attacking the breakers.

I have reflected on how I would react to the options, if I was diagnosed with cancer with a poor outcome based on what I saw with the way Celeste's cancer was handled. Knowing the cancer would not be cured, treatment might or might not extend the duration of life, my inclination as of now, based on what I saw Celeste go through, is that I would refuse treatment.

I would look at some alternatives. I am impressed with the vitamin C outcomes along with other vitamins. Diet may be the strongest defense we have in the way of life choices. I would be willing to eat most anything if there was good evidence that it would be helpful. The description that would apply in my case, I would put most anything in my mouth that was small enough and would swallow anything I could chew.

Chemical therapy may reduce tumors and reduce cancer cells, along with normal cells, but cure is evasive. Chemo and all cancer treatments use toxic chemicals that harm the body and most people dying of cancer likely are dying from the chemical treatment, which may be a quicker death than the show death of cancer itself. Celeste's heart and kidneys were so damaged by the chemical treatments, especially the last treatments, that she actually died of heart failure. The kidneys could not separate the excess potassium out of her body and as a consequence, the high potassium in her blood spiked to damage her heart. We were warned by the cardiology people that spiking of the potassium to a reading of 7.0mmol/L would be dangerous to her heart. Her potassium reached this level on at least three occasions that we were aware.

THE ENGLISH LANGUAGE USED TO WRITE A BOOK

> The most interesting information comes from children,
> for they tell all they know and then stop.
>
> ---Mark Twain

Homographs are words of like spelling but with more than one meaning.

A homograph that is also pronounced differently is a heteronym.

The people responsible for the English language obviously got bored easily. Consider what they did to us!

1) The bandage was *wound* around the *wound*.
2) The farm was used to *produce produce*
3) The dump was so full that it had to *refuse* more *refuse*.
4) We must *polish* the *Polish* furniture.
5) He could *lead*if he would get the *lead* out.
6) The soldier decided to *desert* his dessert in the *desert*.
7) Since there is no time like the *present*, he thought it was time to *present* the *present*.
8) A *bass* was painted on the head of the *bass* drum.
9) When shot at, the *dove dove *into the bushes.
10) I did not *object* to the *object*.
11) The insurance was *invalid* for the *invalid*.
12) There was a *row* among the oarsmen about how to *row*.

13) They were too *close* to the door to *close* it.
14) The buck *does* funny things when the *does* are present.
15) A seamstress and a *sewer* fell down into a *sewer* line.
16) To help with planting, the farmer taught his *sow* to *sow*.
17) The *wind* was too strong to *wind* the sail.
18) Upon seeing the *tear* in the painting I shed a *tear*.
19) I had to *subject* the *subject* to a series of tests.
20) How can I *intimate* this to my most *intimate* friend?

Let's face it - English is a crazy language.

There is no egg in eggplant, nor ham in hamburger; neither apple nor pine in a pineapple.

English muffins weren't invented in England or French fries in France. Sweetmeats are candies while sweetbreads, which aren't sweet, are meat.

We take English for granted. But if we explore its paradoxes, we find that

quicksand can work slowly, boxing rings are square and a guinea pig is neither from Guinea nor is it a pig

And why is it that writers write but fingers don't fing, grocers don't groce and hammers don't ham? If the plural of tooth is teeth, why isn't the plural of booth, beeth? One goose, 2 geese. So, one moose, 2 meese?

One index, 2 indices? Doesn't it seem crazy that you can make amends but not one amend?

If you have a bunch of odds and ends and get rid of all but one of them, what do you call it?

If teachers taught, why didn't preachers praught?

If a vegetarian eats vegetables, what does a humanitarian eat?

In what language do people recite at a play and play at a recital?

Ship by truck and send cargo by ship! Have noses that run and feet that smell.

How can a slim chance and a fat chance be the same, while a wise man and a wise guy are opposites?

You have to marvel at the unique lunacy of a language in which your house can burn up as it burns down, in which you fill in a form by filling it out and in which, an alarm goes off by going on.

English was invented by people, not computers, and it reflects the creativity of the human race, which, of course, is not a race at all.

That is why, when the stars are out, they are visible, but when the lights are out, they are invisible.

One more consideration! Why doesn't 'Buick' rhyme with 'quick'? AND if a male sheep is called a ram and a donkey is called an ass, why is a ram-in-the-ass called a goose?

LEXOPHILES

These are not original

Education is not just filling the basket, it is lighting a fire!

Don't spell part backwards, it's a trap.

When two egotists meet, its an I for an I.

I wondered why the baseball was getting bigger, then it hit e.

Does the name Pavlov ring a bell?

Police were called to a day care where a three-year-old was resisting a rest.

Did you hear about the guy whose whole left side was cut off?

He's all right now.

I can't believe I got fired from the calendar factory. All I did was take a day off.

Corduroy pillows are making headlines.

The roundest knight at King Arthur's round table was Sir Cumference.

To write with a broken pencil is pointless.

If a clock is hungry, does it go back four seconds?

When fish are in schools, they sometimes take debate.

If a short psychic broke out of jail, you'd have a small medium at large.

A thief who stole a calendar got twelve months.

Most people are shocked when they find out how incompetent I am as an electrician.

A thief fell and broke his leg in wet cement. He became a hardened criminal.

Thieves who steal corn from a garden could be charged with stalking.

We'll never run out of math teachers because they always multiply.

When the smog lifts in Los Angeles, U.C.L.A.

I was addicted to the hokey pokey; but, thankfully, I turned myself around.

The math professor went crazy with the blackboard. He did a number on it.

When an actress saw her first strands of gray hair, she thought she'd dye.

The professor discovered that her theory of earthquakes was on shaky ground.

I've just written a song about tortillas; actually, it's more of a rap.

The dead batteries were given out free of charge.

If you take a laptop for a run, you could jog your memory.

A dentist and a manicurist fought tooth and nail.

A bicycle can't stand alone; it is two tired.

When she told me I was average, she was just being mean.

A will is a dead giveaway.

Time flies like an arrow; fruit flies like a banana.

A backward poet writes inverse.

In a democracy it's your vote that counts; in feudalism, it's your Count that votes.

A chicken crossing the road: poultry in motion.

If you don't pay your exorcist, you can get repossessed.

With her marriage, she got a new name and a dress.

Show me a piano falling down a mine shaft, and I'll show you A-flat miner.

Don't trust atoms; they make up everything.

The guy who fell onto an upholstery machine was fully recovered.

A grenade fell onto a kitchen floor in France, resulted in Linoleum Blownapart.

Your debt will stay with you if you can't budge it.

Local Area Network in Australia: The LAN down under.

He broke into song because he couldn't find the key.

A calendar's days are numbered.

A lot of money is tainted: 'Taint yours, and 'taint mine.

A boiled egg is hard to beat.

A successful diet is the triumph of mind over platter.

He had a photographic memory, which was never developed.

A plateau is a high form of flattery.

When you've seen one shopping center you've seen a mall.

I'd tell you a chemistry joke, but I know I wouldn't get a reaction.

If you jump off a Paris bridge, you are in Seine.

Bakers trade bread recipes on a knead to know basis.

Santa's helpers are subordinate clauses.

Acupuncture: a jab well done.

SAYINGS

1. Do not regret growing older; it is a privilege denied to many.
2. Live your life and forget your age.
3. I have seen better days, but also worse.
4. I don't have everything I want but all I need.
5. I wake up with aches and pains, but I wake up which is important.
6. My life is not perfect but good.
7. Spending time on children is more important than spending money on children.
8. If you are at peace, you are living in the present.
9. Take care of your thoughts when alone, take care of words when with people.
10. Nature, cheaper than therapy.
11. Live simply, expect little, give much.
12. If you have integrity, nothing else matters; if you don't have integrity, nothing else matters. ….. Ben Franklin.
13. The pathetic consists in the detail of little events.
14. Education is not just filling the basket; it is lighting a fire.
15. Get your facts first, then you can distort them as you lease.
16. The most interesting information comes from children, for they tell all they know and then stop …. Mark Twain.
17. The pathetic almost always consists in the detail of little events. …. Mark Twain
18. A good thing about being old, not much peer pressure.
19. If you have integrity, nothing else matters; If you don't have integrity, nothing else matters. …. Ben Franklin.
20. Life is short, break the rules. Forgive quickly, laugh uncontrollably, and never regret anything that makes you smile. …. Mark Twain

21. Going to church does not make you a Christian any more than standing in a garage makes you a car.
22. People will hate you, rate you, shake you, and break you. How strong you stand is what makes you.
23. Hopes and dreams are not fulfilled because someone did not take the first step.
24. Out of clutter, find Simplicity. From discord, find Harmony. In the middle of difficulty lies Opportunity.
25. The art of medicine consists in amusing the patient while nature cures the disease. …. Voltaire (1694-1778).
26. Have a caring heart, a smile that never fades, and a touch that never hurts.
27. Work is about a search for daily meaning as well as daily bread.
28. The Lord said to the brethren, go and celebrate. A monk copied "celibate". (For that, many have struggled with themselves far too long!).
29. Many things will work again, if unplugged for a while, including people.
30. Commitment is an act, not a word.
31. There is nothing harder than the softness of indifference.
32. There is only one thing worse than camping; camping with other people.
33. When holding an elephant by the hind leg and it wants to un, let it go.
34. The less people know, the more stubbornly they know it.
35. Facts are stubborn things: and whatever may be our wishes, our inclinations, or the dictates of our passions, they cannot alter the state of facts and evidence. …. John Adams.
36. Give me the senility to forget people I never liked in the first place.

CPSIA information can be obtained
at www.ICGtesting.com
Printed in the USA
JSHW081246231122
33645JS00002B/13